BASIC GROUPWORK

Second Edition

Tom Douglas

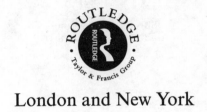

London and New York

First published 1978
by Tavistock Publications Limited
Reprinted 1988, 1990, 1993, 1995 by Routledge
Second edition 2000 by Routledge
11 New Fetter Lane, London EC4P 4EE

Simultaneously published in the USA and Canada
by Routledge
29 West 35th Street, New York, NY 10001

Routledge is an imprint of the Taylor & Francis Group

© 2000 Tom Douglas

Typeset in Times by
M Rules

Printed and bound in Great Britain by
Clays Ltd, St Ives PLC

British Library Cataloguing in Publication Data
A catalogue record for this book is available from the British Library

Library of Congress Cataloging in Publication Data
Douglas, Tom
Basic groupwork/Tom Douglas – 2nd edition
p. cm
Includes bibliographical references and index.
1. Social group work.   I. Title
HV45 .D66 2000 99-057246
361.4–dc21

ISBN 0 415 22479 9 (hbk)
ISBN 0 415 22480 2 (pbk)

BASIC GROUPWORK
Second Edition

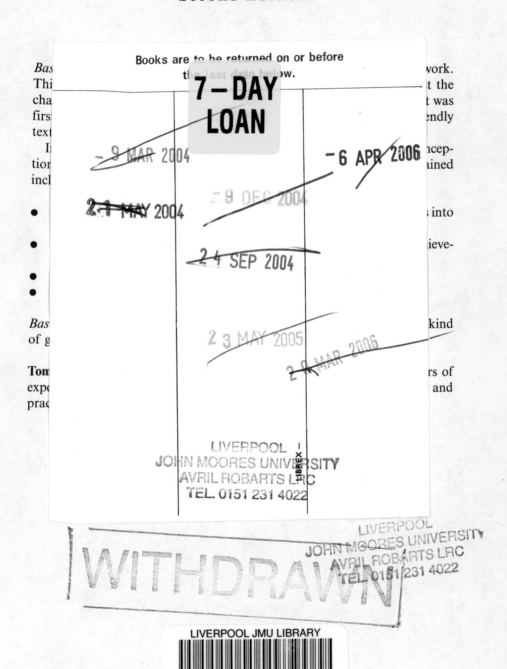

Bas . . . . work.
Thi . . . . t the
cha . . . . t was
firs . . . . endly
text . . . .

I . . . . ncep-
tior . . . . ined
incl . . . .

- . . . . into
- . . . . ieve-
- . . . .
- . . . .

Bas . . . . kind
of g . . . .

Tom . . . . rs of
expe . . . . and
prac . . . .

TO SHIRLEY
AS EVER

CONTENTS

PREFACE

Interest in the use of groups has burgeoned over the past twenty years, as witness the vast increase in the amount of literature about groups and groupwork which has been produced. A great deal of that change has occurred in ways which were hardly foreseen in 1978 when *Basic Groupwork* was first published.

However, one thing has become increasingly clear over that period, which is that my impression, strong even in 1976–7, that it is difficult to learn how to work in and with groups in an effective manner, is more than justified. I think there are several reasons for this, and the strongest is that there is still a powerful concentration on individuality in the Western world – which, despite the fact that we are born into and live and work during most of our lives in groups of some form or other, is not really surprising. For we are always conscious of the fact that we exist and indeed that we know of things outside of ourselves only through the sensory inputs we receive and the interpretations we place upon those inputs.

But we are social creatures, despite the attempts some of us make to keep apart and distant from others. The influence of the groups we inhabit has a great and lasting effect upon our behaviour, and also on the way we think – not to say *what* we think. Such influences are not unknown to us but we tend to think of them as 'natural' – that is, that they are just part of 'what is' – and for a great deal of the time we tend to ignore them or ascribe their influence to other factors such as fate. But we do see people who appear to have ideas and opinions different from those we hold, who seem to follow different belief systems and who have different codes of behaviour. We know, when we think about it, that these different behaviours stem largely from the fact that such people belong to social groupings which are significantly different from those to which we belong. But somehow, to make that connection backwards, as it were, to see the group pressures and influences which have given us our belief systems, seems to be much more difficult. Perhaps because those systems are ours they are therefore 'natural', which means in effect that we did not consciously strive to acquire them. They just grew.

The many major changes in British society since the first edition of *Basic Groupwork* was written would in any case have necessitated a revision of that text if it were to be relevant for groupworkers in the third millennium AD. For instance, in 1977 it was possible to write a book about working with people which made only brief reference to the effect that ethnic minorities made on society. Statistics for 1996 show that ethnic minorities form 6 per cent of a population of 58.2 million, and it is not surprising that attitudes towards such a substantial proportion have had to undergo some radical revision and indeed legislation.

Most groupwork then was founded either on a leisure approach or on the model of therapy, often based on some form of psychodynamic theoretical underpinnings. This was not surprising; the great burgeoning of the use of groups in all the many manifestations that have occurred since was in reality just beginning.

Other great changes in society which have occurred are the greater personal freedom that individuals now have to express their individuality in all manner of ways, the more liberal attitudes towards sexual behaviour, and the freeing of many from the restraints of traditional forms of behaviour. The social standing of women has also changed. But amongst all these liberalizing changes, other changes have not been so beneficial. For instance, there has been the creation of what the press has called an 'underclass', which in effect means that there are many who have grown up without being able to obtain satisfying work. Many forms of poverty still exist; for instance, some estimates say that roughly 4.5 million children are being brought up in conditions of poverty, and many people are homeless. Moreover, the society which believed in a job for life has had to come to terms with the idea that this form of personal security is not available to many any more.

There is also the fact that many people in our society are less prepared to accept the dictates of authority. More are inclined to seek redress and compensation for wrongs which they believe have been inflicted upon them by the unjust and unfair behaviour of those with power, and indeed powerlessness and the consequent efforts of some to redress this imbalance, along with efforts to combat discrimination, have become widespread.

Given that what individuals bring into groups are themselves and that those selves have been formed by the society in which they have grown up, acting upon genetic endowment, then these developments have inevitably resulted in changes in the way groups can be formed and in the ways their members can be expected to react in them. For instance, the issues which are to be found in the society at large can inevitably be found in the smaller social units which are groups – simple things like whether members should be allowed to smoke, or complex factors like the issues of race, sexual orientation, power and different value systems.

Whereas the basic ways in which groups operate are still and always will be the same, and indeed many of the basic needs and interests of members are the same, the changes which have occurred in society require that group-workers need to take cognizance of what has occurred in terms of changes both in general and of specific belief systems, and changes in the desires of those who become, or are compelled to become, members of groups.

All these changes will, I hope, be reflected in this book in the way that groupworkers and group members will be offered help in using the ubiquitous group processes. But one other change at least is worth mentioning here, which is the emphasis that modern theorists place upon the individual's ability to think on and reflect upon his/her behaviour and, with or without help, to bring about change. There is a much stronger and more prevalent belief now than in the 1970s that what are demonstrably present are an individual's behaviour and his/her and our consciousness of it, and what are not present are the sources of that behaviour. Thus it is only logical that we should attempt to work with what we have and not so much with what we assume to have caused it.

Given that many are not wholly aware of their behaviour patterns and how they affect others, that equally many will not have thought about the matter at all or even want to, then the approach that reveals to them how their behaviour appears to others, followed by the offering of information and guidance, may well give them for the first time some ability consciously to control aspects of their behaviour.

It boils down to the fact that whether the behaviour in question is one of a great lack of social competence through lack of opportunity to learn or behaviour which is asocial, unless the individual becomes aware of it and then decides to do something about it, very little real change will actually occur, or if it does occur, it will not endure. In simple terms, the only lasting changes which can be made in human behaviour have to come from the individuals who are targets of change. This is usually summed up either in terms of 'public conformity' for change, which is brought about by the application of outside pressure, or 'private acceptance' for the change, which is brought about by an individual's desire to change. Changed behaviour of the former type tends to revert to previous patterns when the pressure to conform is lifted, while the latter type stands a greater chance of becoming integrated.

Among the younger generation in Western societies the exponential growth of interest in and use of computers has re-emphasized individualization and social separation. The relationship between individual and machine has taken away some of the relationship system which existed between individuals, and, as psychologists are beginning to assert, the communication between individuals via the Internet and other electronic systems is not, and cannot be, the same as that in a face-to-face contact with a real, live person. The contact may be 'virtual' but it is not real.

Groups have always been used from earliest times for any sort of task which required more than could be given to it by one person alone. Equally, when the same information has had to be distributed to a large number of people in a short time, it has always been possible to do an efficient job by gathering into the same place all those, or significantly large groups of those, who are to be recipients. The family, kin groups, friendship groups bound by blood ties or by liking have always existed, but the salient point is that these groups have always been regarded as 'natural' – that is, they arose as it were spontaneously as a response to situations in which individuals found themselves. Few, until fairly recently, considered that such groups were susceptible of being analysed to see why and how they performed their functions so successfully. They just did!

I have argued elsewhere (Douglas, 1983) that an analysis of these apparently spontaneously occurring groups can reveal how they work and that these revelations can form the basis for an understanding of how groups which are not 'spontaneous' but which are created by individuals in order to gain the advantages that they believe can accrue from co-operative combination, can best be created and operate. It comes down to the fact that given that we live in a social environment – that is, in the presence of others – then groups have a considerable influence on the ways we behave and on what we believe to be right and wrong. So if it is possible to create group systems to take advantage of the influence factors which we know to exist in spontaneous groups, we would be very foolish not to do so.

There is another reason for trying to locate and understand the processes which operate in groups, which is that we are all members of many groups. Some of these we know have a decided effect upon our patterns of thinking and behaviour, but there are many others where the influence is hidden from our awareness of it. But such influences could surely be brought into consciousness if we only knew more about the ways in which such groups work. The advantage is clear: where we once operated under influences of which we were not wholly aware, with understanding there would arise the possibility of choice either to accept the influence or not to do so. What group influences drive individuals to ethnic cleansing, to racial violence and other forms of prejudice-loaded behaviour? Such hatreds are almost always instigated by those who make continual selective reference to historical events and are maintained by group pressures which may be understood by others at a superficial level but not at all at the more powerful hidden depths.

I have based what I have written here, as I did in 1976–7, on what I have done over the years in group situations; on my research into how groups work; and on the themes that I have found myself repeating over and over again to those with whom I have worked to generate knowledge of groups and some skill in working with them. Once again I have not attempted to write an academic text full of references to research projects. Rather, I have aimed to present as directly and forthrightly as I could a basic approach to groups and groupwork. One of the reason for choosing to do it this way is that I have been approached by more individuals concerned and perplexed by the complex and apparently diverse and contradictory ideas expressed in texts on group behaviour and on groupwork than on any other problem associated with the subject. Whole new languages have been created about group dynamics, and issues which are at best almost amorphous and changing have appeared as concrete certainties. All this tends to obscure what the individual who wishes to know how he/she might best set up and run, say, a neighbourhood watch scheme believes should be available in such texts. Because groups are to be found everywhere in all societies, the language used to discuss them and to learn about them should be the language of everyday life. It avails us little to talk about common experiences which, while they might not be obvious, are nevertheless there, in words which only serve to prevent learning taking place.

In a very real sense, and despite the fact that the actual understanding of precisely how groups work is still lacking, many people do seem to be much more aware of the uses to which groups can be put in achieving a wide variety of aims, some of which we will look at later. But I would still hazard an informed guess that unless at least some of the members of any group are professional group organizers or individuals with some considerable experience of group formation and use who have also thought about their activities in a serious and reflective way, not too many of these group members know or could explain why groups can be so successful in helping people achieve such a wide variety of aims, except in the broadest terms such as support and the effectiveness of numbers.

The purpose of this book, then, is to help individuals look afresh at their own experiences in groups and to assist them to organize those experiences in such a fashion that they can begin to understand rather more clearly what goes on in group situations. No book can by itself show anyone how to work effectively in and with groups. To do so needs at least some practical on-the-spot supervision by someone with a good working knowledge of groupwork and some skills as a teacher. But at least some of the problems relating to understanding group behaviour can be presented here and then it can be shown how that understanding can be used as the basis upon which practical skills can be founded.

The structure of the book is simple: it follows a logical linear progression. The first half will show how groups work:

- It will examine the many different forms which groups take.
- It will then question why there are so many forms, and show that it is because they are found to be successful in meeting and answering some basic human needs.
- The book will look at the characteristics of potential group members, especially their belief systems and desires. These are, after all, the beginnings and constituents of any group, and it is logical that we should look at the properties which they bring into any group and, briefly, how they acquired them.

- Then we will look at how these properties, operating in the restricted social space within a group, generate what are called the group processes: the consistent patterns of behaviour which the interaction of group members tends to produce.
- All groups operate in an environment, and the constraints which this and other factors place upon any group, combined with the acts of leadership and behaviour of members, are the main elements in the formation of the group processes.
- There are several different kinds of leadership ranging from directive to enabling and guiding; we will look at these here.

The second half of the book will follow the general process of conceptualizing a group, through turning ideas into action to the running of a group and the responsibility involved, and then to the ways in which groups end, carry on or are transformed into a different group or other entity.

Finally, the last chapter examines some ideas about the knowledge and skills of groupwork and how they might be acquired.

I think it is appropriate here to make clear what I mean by 'basic' and also by 'groupwork'. There are two principal meanings to each term, thus:

- Groupwork is what groups do, i.e. the work that groups perform as an integrated unit.
- Groupwork is also the work that specific individuals perform with groups of people in, for instance, the creation of groups and as leaders, members, convenors and enablers, etc.
- Basic groupwork comprises the fundamental functions of groups, some of which are found in all groups, and is most usually referred to as 'group processes'.
- Basic groupwork also comprises the essential skills and knowledge which are the absolute essentials for any individual seeking to create, adapt and work with groups most usually for beneficial ends.

Groups are not the prerogative of professional helpers. They are to be seen as a means of support and help for any one who cares to try to form, or work within, a group.

Many things have changed in British society since *Basic Groupwork* was first published, and the text has now been extensively revised and rewritten to bring it up to date. However, the processes by which groups develop their particular methods of functioning have not changed. The changes, both of emphasis and in kind, are rather to some of the components that individuals bring into them, based upon changes in belief systems and desires.

The original text was based on the premise that *all* groups developed the same processes, provided that they existed long enough. This is still indubitably true. These processes are inherent in the formation of any group as a social system and are thus a basic, generic characteristic of groups. It now seems accepted that because a group – any group – is a microcosm of the behavioural and belief patterns of the communities from which its members come, that the group will reproduce the social patterns current in those communities, though not always in the same proportions or intensities. Because these patterns are usually clearly exposed to observation only when they occur within the confined social space of a group, they become much more visible than they were in the larger community, where they tended to be masked by familiarity and by our tendency to concentrate on individual behaviour until group behaviour is exposed by a given set of circumstances.

Small groups have a catalytic effect in making very visible interactions, behavioural patterns, rules, norms, standards, values, traditions and the essential belief systems of their individual members. It has therefore been my endeavour to accommodate these ideas in the rewriting and to counter to some extent the original edition's over-emphasis on the specialist/authority forms of leadership images of the groupworker.

ACKNOWLEDGEMENTS

In the 1978 version of this text I acknowledged my great indebtedness to all those students, ex-students, colleagues and friends who had allowed me to quote from their records of groups. That indebtedness still stands. But now I must add to it my grateful thanks to all those, who, over the past twenty years, have given me access to their work, their successes and their problems in so many more areas of groupwork than I originally had experience of, and thus have helped me to reformulate some of my ideas of what actually constitutes basic groupwork. I owe a special debt to my friend and colleague David Warren-Holland for his invaluable help.

Part I

HOW GROUPS WORK

1

A VERY DIVERSE FAMILY

The range of group forms

Ay, in the catalogue ye go for men;
As hounds, and greyhounds, mongrels, spaniels, curs,
Shoughs, water-rugs, and demi-wolves are clept
All by the name of dogs: the valu'd file
Distinguishes the swift, the slow, the subtle,
The housekeeper, the hunter, every one
According to the gift which bounteous Nature
Hath in him clos'd; whereby he does receive
Particular addition, from the bill
That writes them all alike; and so of men.

William Shakespeare, *Macbeth* III.i.11

What Shakespeare implied about men and dogs is equally true about human groups: the apparent variety is immense and yet they all derive from a common stock. Even a cursory look around society will reveal an amazing number of seemingly different groups. There are groups formed for protection, such as neighbourhood watch schemes; for the removal of social nuisance behaviour, e.g. groups for those who offend by being racist, sexist or violent, or who sexually or physically abuse children or are guilty of rape; groups to exert pressure on decision-making bodies so as to try to obtain for a specific area amenities and facilities such as crossings for schoolchildren; literacy groups to enable those who cannot read or write to obtain adequate skills; groups which are set up to help those who are or who care for individuals with illnesses and handicaps like cystic fibrosis or mental illness or strokes; there are groups set up as special and specific therapy units for all manner of different problems, illnesses and complaints; there are groups which arise to meet the problems of those suffering from some particular need like Weight-Watchers and Alcoholics Anonymous; there are fitness groups, leisure groups, training groups, special-interest groups; learning groups and classes of all sorts; work groups, clubs, societies, issues groups, groups for justice for some end or other; sponsor groups and groups for specific communities, ethnic minorities and so on – the list is endless. But, as I hope to show quite clearly, most groups, whatever their kind or origin, have more in common than they have in difference. However, at this point I am concerned with their differences.

3

DIFFERENCES

Perhaps the simplest and most usually offered distinction between groups is that which divides them into 'natural' or 'created' groups. The distinction is more apparent than real, but it is of immense psychological importance. Individuals have an innate suspicion of 'created' groups on the grounds that they are artificial, whereas what is perceived as a 'natural' group, such as a family or a friendship group, is more acceptable because its origins lie in the history of any particular culture and it does not have the appearance of having been set up deliberately and with intent.

A natural group is one which arose to meet a particular purpose, which essentially has to be one which is other than that of the creation itself. In other words, it arose because there was a task to perform which could best be met by a number of individuals working together, but in which no great emphasis was placed upon the way in which the group existed as a definable social system. Indeed, this aspect would rarely be acknowledged at all. Created groups, by contrast, are those which are brought into being by virtue of the conscious intent of one or more people to create a group to meet some specific purpose. Such people have more or less understanding of the properties which groups develop and of their apparent usefulness in achieving certain kinds of ends.

In natural groups, the group form is a very minor consideration in the major need to generate a kind of organization of the resources necessary to meet an urgent need; in the second type of group, the group's creation in order to use its functional processes is an intentional process which is much more cognizant of the actual processes that operate within groups.

In a sense the dichotomy natural/created is confusing. What is probably much closer to reality is the degree of consciousness of the dynamics of groups and of the intent of the originators of groups to use that knowledge. In all probability the only truly natural group is the family when it is based around the production and protection of children, and their nurture. It is natural because in some form or other it has always existed, and because without some form of long-term protection no human infant would survive. But even here, as we shall see, the family unit can be composed in a variety of different ways, as witness the rise in the number of sole-parent families over the past twenty years.

So the process by which a groupworker seeks to make the members of the group aware of the dynamics – the processes – of a group so that they become available to be used is one of developing an attention to and conscious awareness of those processes, in the same way that individuals interested in painting can be brought to see colour and form in a way that most people do not.

THE GROUP AS CONTEXT AND AS INSTRUMENT

A very important distinction between groups is the one drawn between the group as context and the group as instrument. Now, this is a piece of jargon which represents a distinction that many people find very hard to grasp, although it represents a very real difference, one which is more than just a difference in the way the group happens to be run and is a much more fundamental distinction of belief about the way in which human beings can change their thinking and behaviour patterns.

A group can be set up in which the basic aim is that each individual member works with the leadership in achieving that individual's own personal goals. The rest of the group form a background to this work and each takes this position of interaction with the leadership in turn. Many therapy groups are run on exactly these lines. When this occurs, the group is said to be *the context*. Other groups are set up in which the leadership try to establish a situation in which all the members come to trust one another sufficiently to see the advantages of working together as a unit. In other words, they assume responsibility for the running of the group. The leadership is not now unduly dominant as the members exercise the power and the influence they have learned to grasp for their mutual benefit. In this case the group itself – that is, the sum total of its members and leadership acting as a unit – has become *the instrument* of achievement.

However, if the ideas of context and instrument appear difficult, a simpler version is at hand in the form of style of leadership. Briefly, there are three main points on the range of leadership styles. They are usually defined as *directive*, i.e. leader-oriented; *enabling* or *facilitative*, i.e. group oriented; and *mutual*. Very few groups are actually found operating as pure forms of these salient points. Most are combinations of the main forms, according to their appropriateness to the stage which a group has reached in its life. But before we look at the possible complications, let us look briefly at the 'pure' forms, as we will consider the nature of leadership in more detail in Chapter 5.

Groups which benefit from a directive leadership are usually those where the actual resources of the group members are of secondary importance to those exercised by the leadership. Such groups are those in which the understanding and knowledge of the leadership is essential in guiding the group members, explaining, offering information to which the members had no previous access, revealing the consequences of particular behavioural patterns which were being avoided or which may never have been previously considered, and in general applying knowledge on a wider, more substantial scale to the kinds of predicaments and problems possessed by the group's members. In system terminology, most of the energy, input and control of response comes from the leadership. This does not mean that the contribution of the members is of no importance, or there would be no advantage in their being members of such a group and group members' problems could just as well be

5

dealt with on a one-to-one basis. Members learn about their own personal patterns of problems from being present as the similar problems of fellow members are dealt with, and then they work with the leadership in the context of the group when their turn arrives and provide learning opportunities for their fellows in turn. Alternatively, the leadership may work with the total group membership by a process of involving them by direct approaches and by setting tasks and exposing what is going on in the group.

Enabling and facilitative leadership is a process of encouragement by which the leadership sets out with the basic intent of showing the members of a group what resources they possess and the ways in which these can be used in dealing with the business for which the group was established, and supporting them while they learn the ropes. In some ways this form of leadership may be just as controlling as directive leadership. The essential difference is that pure directive leadership is promulgated on the assumption of retaining control of the group's processes during the whole of the group's existence. Facilitative leadership, on the other hand, uses directive techniques with the intent of teaching by demonstration and controlled experience that the control and use of the group's resources is available to group members and the power and skill in their use can be developed. This essential difference may in the end be located in a different understanding of how people can change their behaviour. In the latter the belief rests on the assumption that 'true' change – that is, change which 'sticks' – can only come from the individual's willingness to change. This is usually referred to as the 'private acceptance' of change. Directive leadership seems to be founded in the assumption that the problems some people face can be resolved only by the application of external expertise and by their being constrained to follow certain well-defined paths.

In essence, mutual groups are self-help groups, a combinatorial exercise in which individuals with the same or similar concerns band together in order to obtain satisfaction of those concerns which they have usually found unattainable when operating on their own. Such groups are often generated by some of those who become their members; they are essentially numerically supportive, and leadership is of the order of a committee structure, either self-imposed or elective, depending on the perception members have of the value and worth of individual members in exercising some rights of leadership. Some such groups are brought into existence at the suggestion of professional workers, who take some responsibility for helping the group get off the ground, but take no hand in its direction. They may remain available to be consulted if the group so wishes when advice and information would be helpful.

Where people are facing a situation which has the potential to bring about large changes in their accustomed lifestyle, then fear of the unknown, anxiety about the possible consequences, and worry about whether their coping behaviours will prove to be adequate frequently occur. At such a point in life, one individual may well be very pleased to meet someone who has passed through this stage as well as a number of others who are just going through it. In the first instance, the individual is presented with a person who has undergone a group experience and apparently survived and benefited from it. Such a person can talk from personal experience about what happened to others who are going through a similar experience. Such an individual carries a high level of credibility and can help to expose others to different viewpoints and also to different ways of trying to cope.

Within limits, more people means more ideas, and thus the possibility that ways of approaching a problem or a predicament which individual members of a group had not thought of for themselves can be presented for their consideration and eventual use. It is these factors of experience and the production of alternative ideas which can be successfully exploited by groups with a large element of self-help about them. For instance, it would seem that for individuals whose behaviour is regarded as asocial, and those who are addicted to drugs, say, what works is that they are given the chance to live in a community where *they* make the rules and *they* enforce them – a democracy in which each member can come to realize that s/he is responsible for his/her own behaviour and also for the behaviour of the community as a whole.

A large number of groups currently in existence have a form of leadership which is exercised by more than one person – that is, co-leadership or partnership. In such cases the individual leaders may not only have different styles on the range of directive/enabling, but also attend to different areas of the group process. For example, one may be attentive to the group's performance of their allotted task while another will be devoted to the interpersonal relationships of the members. Leaders may also act as role models of particular areas of human relationships, e.g. male/female; black/white; and so on.

As I hope to show later, several forms of leadership may occur in a single group over its duration in order to meet the assessed needs of the group at a particular time. This can only occur, however, if the leadership is not wholly grounded in the assumption that only one form or kind of leadership is appropriate. Such a decision, usually based upon the whole-hearted acceptance of a particular dogma concerning human behaviour, renders the leadership less flexible in dealing with changes in the group's needs. It must be said, however, with great emphasis, that there are conditions of group members where such an inflexible leadership style is exactly what is required and which confers support and reassurance for members who have little confidence in themselves at that moment in their lives.

DEFINITIONS OF GROUPS

A group can be defined in many ways, such as according to its purpose, its activity, or the field of endeavour in which it is established, and according to

7

the principal theory of human behaviour which motivates the group's direction; to the needs and aims which the group was created to satisfy. We will note some of these approaches to the definition of groups in rather more detail during the course of our explorations. But of much greater immediate need is that we try to explain the enormous spread in the use of groups by looking at the broad principles of why and how they work.

HOW GROUPS WORK

It would seem logical to assume that because groups are so widely used in such a variety of situations, they are actually reasonably successful. On further examination, it is possible to see that groups which operate in certain ways are more successful than others. For instance, those groups which seem to be founded by people who see them as a means to increasing the social power of their members by the simple fact of numbers tend to be successful. Those groups which are based upon supplying a need of their members which cannot be met as well anywhere else and which can therefore draw upon a strong level of commitment are again usually very successful. Those groups which have as their main task the imparting of useful information are also successful, provided that the concept of 'useful' is one derived from the members as much as from the convenors. On the other side of the coin are those groups which are founded with the express purpose of changing behaviour patterns in socially accepted ways; they usually have a fairly tough time in achieving lasting effects.

It is instructive to look at why this is so.

A group is a miniature social system which reflects the behavioural patterns of the society from which its members come. Because it is a small social system, those behaviour patterns, good as well as bad, are available for scrutiny. Once exposed, by the pure fact of occurring in a confined social space in which they can be seen, rather than through any intended confrontational technique, their consequences are available for discussion. Different models of behaviour can be on offer as much from fellow group members as from the group's leadership, with a degree of credibility which is acceptable.

Groups work because human beings have the capacity to process information, to learn from experience and example. Above all, they work because they have some success in allaying suspicion of new and different ideas, in overcoming resistance and anxiety about alternative ways of behaving, and by providing support and understanding from others with similar experiences, difficulties, dilemmas and problems but having different methods of coping. What gives a member of a friendship group the sense of being accepted and able to relax in the company of peers is the same factor which can give the individual member of a group the sense of being freer and well enough

8

supported to try out new, different and potentially more effective ways of thinking and of behaving.

If the group is concerned with increasing the power of its members to pursue their legitimate ends, then the value of numbers is paramount, with the qualification that those numbers, to achieve the best results, should be composed of individuals who are personally involved in achieving those ends and who thus have some considerable degree of commitment to gaining them through the medium of the group. In a sense this success occurs from the realization that there are many tasks which are much more readily achievable with the concerned help of others than can be achieved by individuals acting alone.

If a group is concerned to give support to its members, then once again similar experience in those who form it means that at the very least the members can begin to realize that they are not alone with their problem, whatever it might be. But over and beyond this is the fact that contact with others who have also struggled to deal with similar problems brings the possibility of ideas of new and different approaches in how to cope, as well as the emotional support of being understood in a practical way.

When groups are formed on the basis of some degree of compulsion for those whose behaviour can be described as a matter of public concern, the effectiveness of the groups in question becomes more a matter of how well the group leadership can deal with the resentment and lack of co-operation and commitment which it is highly probable exists in the members. Moreover, the group's members may well have been through similar situations before and therefore have become 'group sophisticates' who are quite able to work the 'system'.

I think we can now look at three interesting factors involved in the process of groupwork: commitment, probability and consequences.

Commitment

It is simple enough to see that where potential group members have a vested interest in a group which they hope will deliver something they desire, one of the major factors of group success is already present. Commitment equals energy, and energy is what is required if a group – any group – is to succeed. The members may not know how to harness that commitment and energy, and that lack may well cause the group to founder. But essentially such a lack is what can be supplied by an experienced groupworker who has seen how such commitment can be guided into fulfilling a group's objectives.

One problem with commitment is that it cannot develop in a particular group unless the individuals concerned are able to believe with some degree of confidence that the group in question is able to deliver what they desire, or at least a substantial part of it. This is a simple enough situation of costs and rewards which in practice is often not quite so simple because it is complicated by matters like desperation, past experience, caution and igno-rance. Where they have a choice, individuals will usually want to assess for themselves whether any commitment, not just in energy but in time and in alternative uses of that time and energy, is going to be worth making. Much of the early stages of a group's life can be devoted to providing some evi-dence, evidence that the members will accept, that the group offers some valid probability that it can and will achieve most of what the members want. It will be essential later in this book to deal with the preparation of individ-uals to become members of successful groups. Time is often the essential factor here, and also of great importance is the process of 'holding' the group until, from personal experience of its functioning, the group members begin to become aware of what the group has to offer. If that awareness is of a rea-sonable probability of success, the commitment to achieve it will usually be made available.

Groups can develop quite warm, friendly atmospheres in which members feel comfortable and accepted in their membership. This is often a very good thing, but most groups have a specified time in which to achieve their goals, after which members should be able to take away with them what they have gained inside the group and apply it in their lives outside it. In one sense, nearly all groups have to develop the commitment of their members, then use that commitment to invest energy in the group to achieve its goals. But in the process they have also to ensure that the group's members consolidate and integrate whatever it is that they have benefited from while in the group. Many follow-up reports of apparently successful groups show that once their members are deprived of the support of the group, the pressures, which may have been the original reason for their need of the group, reassert themselves in the ex-member's life to the gradual erosion of the group's benign and developmental influence unless such consolidation has taken place.

Probability

A discussion of the laws of probability is not much in evidence in textbooks on groupwork, or even in social work. Yet like all human endeavours, the processes of groupwork succeed or fail in large measure on the basis of the nature of the assumptions which are made about probability.

All groups are founded on the assumption that they, rather than some other approach to human concerns, will be effective. But whereas probability theory is founded on numbers which can be known and calculated, the assess-ment of probability when dealing with the outcomes of human activity has no such precise basis, and as a result is much less reliable, for the simple reason that human behaviour can change at whim and fancy. However, there is slightly more reason to expect behaviour in a group to be predictable than there is for the individuals who comprise it acting in their more usual and less confining milieu of everyday life.

Thus an essential factor in the effective functioning of groups is concerned with the assessment of the possible negative and positive effects to which the group will be subjected. For this reason, where at all possible those who convene groups try to ensure that as far as they are able to assess them, the potential members they select will bring into the group elements of experience and other resources which will help to make the group work rather than impede its progress. All groupworkers have at some time or another come across groups which have been destroyed simply because one or more members were wholly or largely unsuitable for membership of that particular group. Equally, wholly or partially unsuitable leadership can have the same devastating effect.

As we shall see later when we consider the effects of constraints, both material and environmental elements must also be part of the probability assessment to give the group the best possible start to its existence. As always, probability is a calculation of the odds.

Consequences

An often-quoted assessment of what happens in any form of social intervention is that the major consequences are most usually not what were originally intended. This derives from our inability to calculate with any reasonable degree of accuracy what will happen in the future. This inability, in turn, is the result of the fact that at the time of calculation there are literally hundreds of potential influence factors which we cannot take into account in our reckoning because we simply do not know of their existence. Even if we are aware of them, we are unable to predict the probability of their occurrence, or their possible effect.

The most effective of groups, i.e. those that work, are predicated on the basis of as well-defined parameters as it is possible to achieve. For instance, groups fail because although the aims they set for accomplishment were perhaps very worthy, the groups were established under circumstances which ensured that consequences other than those desired would be much more likely to occur. Prisons, established as centres of re-education and rehabilitation as well as places of confinement, are far less successful in that role than in the informal role of learning centres for the development of criminal skills. The prisoner-based society is in effect the stronger by virtue of being more immediate and numerically more powerful, and also of possessing greater credibility and consistency than the official programmes.

GROUPS ARE SOCIAL INFLUENCE SYSTEMS

The one thing which emerges from this long catalogue of different types of groups and about commitment, probability and consequence is that there

11

are certain very basic and fundamental characteristics which all groups have in common. How should this not be so? They are all composed of human beings who come from similar, though not identical, areas of the same society, and despite their differences of genetic endowment, upbringing, opportunity and choice, they have similar basic needs. Indeed, I would go so far as to say that in those very differences lie most of the resources to which an effective group will strive to have access and to use.

When groups work it is because in the confined social space which is a group, behaviour that is accepted in the society at large becomes more visible to others, and its immediate and long-term consequences become open for scrutiny. Much behaviour is confirmed in society because it is never challenged by any others who are people of significance to the person producing it. When groups work it is because they offer support and encouragement to their members; they offer solidarity, role models, information and, in very crude terms, they offer the effects which only numbers can achieve – that is, being one of many of like mind and having similar problems and predicaments instead of being a solitary struggler with limited coping skills.

2

BEGINNING AT THE BEGINNING
Group members

'Where shall I begin, please your Majesty?'
he asked. 'Begin at the beginning,' the King
said, gravely, 'and go on till you come to the
end: then stop.'
Lewis Carroll, *Alice in Wonderland*, ch. 2

Strangely enough, and despite the king's sage advice, few people when discussing groups start at the beginning. There are several possible reasons for this. One, maybe, is that groups are such an ordinary aspect of everyday life that it becomes easy, though often terribly misleading, to assume that everyone is therefore well versed and indeed knowledgeable about the beginning of groups. Another reason could be that what stems from beginnings is so interesting that people become fascinated by the flower and do not care or even feel the need to know what the seed was like.

I am not implying that no eyes have ever turned towards the beginnings of groups – quite the contrary, but most of those who do examine groups' beginnings are theorists and not those who are involved with working in and with groups of actual people. Most of those who become involved directly with groups seem to start well into the life span of a group, taking on trust that they work – that they are effective in achieving certain outcomes. It seems almost as if such potential group members and workers believe that it is sufficient to accept that ends can be achieved, and the answer to the question WHY? is not often asked for.

In the beginning there must have been some realization of the potential value of groups and of the ways in which these values could be used. So although I appreciate that all introductory writing must appear to some people to be stating the obvious, I think it is necessary to start with the very simple things. For what is obvious to one person is by no means necessarily equally obvious to another, who may have had no apparent reason for even starting to think about it. One of the basic misconceptions which besets human communication is exactly the unchecked assumption that the obvious appears so to all those involved.

The real and absolute beginning of most groups is an idea. Someone somewhere decides that some objective, clear or vague, can be achieved effectively, or sometimes safely, only by a number of people working together, in however a limited manner. This latter point is made quite clear when we look at the enormous range of groups where the number of members is the fundamental element of the group's power, a point we shall have need to return to later.

But ideas sometimes never get turned into action, and so it is that it is usual to aver that the beginning of a group occurs when a number of people are gathered together in a specific location and become aware of each other within that confined space. Of course there are groups, sometimes defined as statistical groups, to which individuals consider themselves to belong who never actually meet on a face-to-face basis. But for our purposes such groups can be left as a peripheral manifestation of group existence, though, as we shall see, they sometimes are responsible for many of the attitudes, beliefs, opinions and traditions which people carry with them during their lives.

So let us begin at the accepted beginning.

A group – any group – is composed of individual members. This is so whether the group is of short or long duration, and whether its membership is static or constantly changing.

Now whatever the manner by which a group came into existence, it has as its basic constituents, with which to perform whatever function it arose to achieve, the beliefs, knowledge, experience, emotions and personalities of those members. They in turn have learned various ways of achieving their personal ends and aims with varying degrees of success or failure. They will also have learned that society, in the form of others with somewhat different beliefs and desires and circumstances, is able to produce levels of frustration or of facilitation of an individual's aims. So some people have learned to trust others in certain ways and in certain situations, and have learned to be suspicious in others. Some can't abide being constrained by rules for which they can see no just application to themselves; still others have found themselves at times overwhelmed by problems for which they find that the coping behaviours they have previously acquired and used prove woefully ineffective; others that by themselves they can make no headway against bureaucratic opinion; others find that their experience has given them the desire to help others avoid or deal with difficulties similar to those which they themselves have experienced.

The list of behaviours which exist, formed from the interaction of genetic endowment and exposure to the process of growing up, living and working in a given society, is absolutely endless. But basic to all the needs, desires, predicaments and problems to which individuals are exposed as a matter of course in the process of just being alive is the fact that this process develops, in each individual, patterns of behaviour which become relatively stable according to how successful they are in helping that individual to cope, to survive, to learn, however good, bad or indifferent may be their quality. Perhaps most important of all in this process, each individual acquires a series of opinions, attitudes and beliefs about him/herself and about what is good or bad, what obligations and rights are involved, all of which together forms what is that individual's belief system. Parts of this system may be very strongly held, almost as inalienable; others may be less strongly entrenched and subject to change, modified by appropriate experience, or even by the presentation and acceptance of factual information different from that upon which they were first based. Also included in this belief system are those desires which the individual would like to achieve, some of which are essentially simple, logical and attainable while others are the stuff of fantasy and plainly inaccessible, though the individual may not be entirely aware of this.

This belief system also includes most of the ideas which the individual has taken on board throughout his/her life, by experience, by contact with others, by imitation and by encouragement and by just being exposed to values and norms. Such values are often quite consistent during the early years, but later the individual is exposed to wider and different situations. Different behaviour patterns will have been seen as the scope to move about increases, as the individual thinks and reflects what has been seen or felt, and almost always some new ideas will replace earlier ones. In some cases opposing ideas will continue to be held, often without the individual being wholly aware of their incongruity. All the factors of culture, of acceptable and unacceptable ways of behaving, will be there, the rules, norms and values, religious and other beliefs, and the codes of moral and ethical conduct.

> In our daily lives we all predict and explain other people's behavior from what we think they know and what we think they want. Beliefs and desires are the explanatory tools of our own intuitive psychology, and intuitive psychology is still the most useful and complete science of behavior there is. To predict the vast majority of human acts – going to the refrigerator, getting on the bus, reaching into one's wallet – you don't need to crank through a mathematical model, run a computer simulation of a neural network, or hire a professional psychologist; you can just ask your grandmother.
>
> (Pinker 1997: 63)

This complex of beliefs and desires is partly unique to the individual and partly shared with others of the same community and age group with whom the individual grew up. Sometimes the two major areas are congruent and exist harmoniously in the one person, and sometimes the two are in conflict in certain areas. One major factor in the creation of belief systems which is of fairly recent origin is the massive increase in information through the medium of television and radio which is available to all in all societies and which contains ideas and knowledge and recorded experience from all over the world brought into each individual's own home, and often reveals aspects of life in distinct contrast to those which are locally acceptable. Thus the parochial nature of most of the commonly held belief systems of a given community now has a powerful and pervasive rival in the form of information technology's offerings, which are international in scope.

Whatever the combination of belief systems and desires which exists in an individual, this is what s/he brings into any group situation and what the group s/he enters has to work with. A group may be able to use what is brought as a resource to help all members of the group; it may be able to help various individuals cope by revealing how others have coped in similar situations; it may be able to show how modifications of the individual's rule system will facilitate existence; it may be able to use what individuals bring to modify behaviour, to gain support for initiatives and aims, and bring about beneficial change. In short, it is from the commonly held belief systems held by the members that what so many groupworkers have described as the 'group processes' derive, and from the differences in those belief systems that change and progress becomes possible.

Of course, such a simple statement is in need of some explanation, which is what this chapter is all about. Thus we will need to look into differences and similarities and show how they can be both advantages and obstacles in groupwork. There are also all the ideas about self-identity, and the use of awareness and intelligence to change moulds of behaviour. Above all, it must be stressed that what we are aiming at is an understanding of the behaviour patterns which people have and which they employ in all situations but which in small groups become patterns that are much more visible. Reciprocally, members of a group can see how others are behaving, and thus comes about the resource system which is fundamental to group process.

Let us start from the social nature of human beings and tackle the idea of individual separateness which tends to drive the need for affiliation and acceptance by 'significant' others and which can be seen as one of the main driving forces that bring about group systems.

Over the years of working with people in groups, I have noted that exercises designed to elicit what most people are afraid of happening nearly always end with an expression in some form or other of the fear of being cut off, of being isolated. This almost universal fear has been expressed in any number of ways from death itself to some situation in which the individual wants, but is unable, to make any kind of contact with fellow human beings. There is here some vague appreciation of the fact, which we all seem to want to avoid recognizing, that in a very simple but direct way we are dependent upon others. Even more important, perhaps, is that we are separate, self-contained biological entities whose only form of contact with others of our species is by means of our senses. The information with which they provide us is essentially interpreted by our brains, giving us a reconstruction of what is outside of ourselves, a kind of 'in-house' virtual reality system. Like all interpretative systems, ours is subject to being idiosyncratic. As Richard Dawkins writes,

The problems raised by subjective consciousness are perhaps the most baffling in all philosophy, and solving them is far beyond my ambition. My suggestion is the more modest one that each species, in each situation, needs to deploy its information about the world in whatever way is most useful for taking action. 'Constructing a model in the head' is a helpful way to express how it is done, and comparing it to virtual reality is especially helpful in the case of humans.

(Dawkins 1989: 283)

There is also the fact that we are not able to get outside of ourselves to see what we might look like to others. But we can monitor the apparent effect that we have upon others and in this way we can begin to develop expectations of how we will be received and add these impressions to the ideas we have of ourselves formed from our inner awareness of ourselves to make up a self-image.

However, in order to get feedback about ourselves from others, the first essential is that others be present. To continue to be in the presence of others, it is also necessary that they at least tolerate our being there, and in order to ensure that, in situations which give free choice of whom one will associate with, we are accepted, it is necessary to behave in ways which will tend to ensure that acceptance. In other words, we need to produce conforming behaviour patterns. If the need to be accepted by any particular group is a very high priority for us, then our efforts to conform will be accordingly that much greater.

This process happens many times over in many different groups. Depending on the degree of freedom which individuals in a particular group have to choose with whom they associate, and to what level of intensity and upon the strength of the need they may feel they have to be accepted, so will those individuals produce what they see and feel to be an appropriate level of conformity. For instance, the small boy who begins to experience people other than his family group who begin to mean a great deal to him may well adopt behavioural patterns which will be accepted by his newly found companions but which, to the consternation of his parents, are more than a little at odds with his previous 'good' behaviour.

To put this very bluntly, any individual who considers that there is a group which s/he would dearly like to join because it appears to offer something which he/she wants is going to do his/her best to conform to the behavioural patterns of that group – which creates a situation in which that group can in effect demand that certain behavioural requirements be fulfilled in return for membership. This is true whether the group in question is a private club like a golf club or a street gang.

To understand this is fundamental, because where there are groups which are founded to produce changes in behavioural patterns but in which the members are compelled to attend, say as a condition of a probation order,

17

then the power of the group to effect the required change has to come from a source other than that of the members' need to belong – unless, of course, such a need can be developed as part of the group's progress.

In other circumstances the power of the group can be defined in terms of what members believe they can get out of it – unless, that is, they are aware of the existence of alternative situations which they believe may be available to meet their needs at less cost. Of course, there is always the possibility that a group can be developed by its members to produce a far more satisfactory return than that which appeared to be available in the beginning. But for this to occur, members have to have some kind of assurance that this is a viable way of proceeding. Such assurance can come from direct experience of seeing such a process occur in a previous group situation or of knowing about such occurrences from fairly reliable sources. There is also the fact that many individuals are quite capable of working out for themselves that the quid pro quo of groups is that it is not likely that you get something for nothing. After all, a group is a tool in the sense that it is a working system which requires energy and commitment if it is to succeed. Such energy and commitment can come from two principal sources: the group members or the group leader. It is usually more effective if it comes from both, but, as we will see later, sometimes one or the other is more effective, for a variety of reasons.

Thus at the expense of being somewhat repetitive, I can state that one of the main sources of influence in a group lies, in the perception of potential and actual members, that it can provide some rewards for a level of costs which those members feel they are prepared to pay. Alternatively, where there is no such perception of direct gain, there may be the perception that not to become a member may incur penalties which stack up to an even greater cost.

Much of the mystique which has surrounded groupwork stems from the employment by practitioners of theories of human behaviour which by and large attempt to show that the causes of that behaviour can be discovered. But what is essentially true about nearly all of these theories is that they are assumptions deductively arrived at and which are non-verifiable except in certain very limited ways.

We may never know for sure how behaviour patterns arise, but we may well be able to see what maintains and sustains them when they are once formed. So we may equally be able to see what is most likely to continue to support them, and also what may be able to change, modify or eliminate them.

But what is 'real' about groups is that they comprise individuals who through time, experience and living have arrived at a point in their lives when they operate as a complex system of manifest and hidden behaviour patterns; of thinking, emoting, feeling and acting. This is 'real' because it can be seen and experienced; it forms what Goffman (1971) called front- and back-stage behaviours. Individuals can think and reflect upon what they know and what they do, about what has happened and what may be about to happen; they have perceptions about the world about them and about the people and things which they find in it; they have response patterns and they are aware of having feelings about people, about themselves and about situations; they can make choices; they have some aptitude for learning and of profiting from experience; they have some controllable influences and some which are uncontrollable; they have developed coping behaviours and good, bad and indifferent adaptations to the circumstances they have encountered; chance and opportunity have played a considerable role in shaping their lives; they have beliefs, traditionally and culturally established; they have limitations and liabilities; parts of their 'equipment' may have fully developed or it may not, largely dependent on chance factors. All this amounts to the fact that they are human beings. But they are also the resources, both potential and actual, which groups can seek to deploy for defined ends. There is nothing remotely mysterious about this.

It must be stressed here that the 'point in their lives' referred to above is not meant to imply an essentially static state for most of us. Because we go on living day by day we meet new experiences which tend to modify some point of the complex of behaviours which is an individual. But by using the term 'point' I am stressing that an individual who arrives in a group is at a particular point in his/her presentation as an individual.

Groups happen all through society. They are just very visible manifestations of ordinary human behaviour, but because of that visibility, the result of operating in what amounts to a small, confined social space, the behaviour of members of groups is open to scrutiny and its consequences made visible, which can lead to support, change, modification or elimination if necessary.

GENETICS, NURTURE AND REFLECTION

It has been customary in the past to state that the earliest group conditioning that any individual receives occurs in the family of origin, and that is still absolutely true. But what has changed is the nature of that early group. A large number of today's children are not born into the traditional elementary family.

Modern advances in genetics, which seems to be on the point of being able to tell which behavioural and other individual characteristics are due to which specific gene, have made it possible for babies to be born who have not been conceived by human copulation but by the processes of in vitro fertilization, artificial insemination by donor, or the use of surrogacy or sperm banks. The genetic endowment of those babies will be different from what might have been expected had the adults who look after them conceived them in the usual way.

Then consider that there is also another possible complexity in that whatever their genetic origin, many babies are reared by adults with whom they have little or no genetic connection. Even more confusing of the relationship patterns is the fact that the adults who rear children exist in various relational combinations, and indeed in many cases in relational isolation. A parenting 'unit' may comprise one, two or more adults, and the children in such a unit may have a variety of genetic and non-genetic relationships with each of them. For instance, in the simplest of patterns children may be adopted, fostered or in care.

Historically there have always been complex relationships and kinship complexities, as witness the many legal battles which have been fought over inheritance and the strenuous attempts to establish degrees of consanguinity. There have been systems like fosterage in Scotland, where children were handed to people outside the family to rear, and similar systems have prevailed in other parts of the world.

So we must separate genetic endowment from the process of child-rearing, and in any case what we are concerned with here are the end products, the inevitable consequences brought about by whatever kind of mixture and rearing has occurred – in a word, the person who arrives in a group.

When individuals are old enough to begin to reflect upon themselves as persons, then the next area of complexity kicks in, which is that there begins to be available to the individual the possibility of effecting change in their behaviour patterns by deliberate intent.

In a society which, like Britain's, has a roughly 6 per cent non-white minority, traditional patterns of child-rearing and of relationships and attitudes have had added to them and been affected in many ways by the traditions and cultural behaviours of ethnic groups which are markedly different. Society has also in the past twenty years witnessed great changes in what are accepted as viable patterns of behaviour.

In sum, what people bring with them into group situations can no longer be defined in the terms of one culture's traditions, if indeed this was ever as true as it was once believed to be.

PROBABILITY AND RISK

Groupworkers and others are used to making some crude estimates of the probability of the success of their efforts in working with people and also about making some elementary calculations of the risks involved. But I am not aware that there has been much attention paid to the probabilities and risks from the point of those who become members of groups. Perhaps there should be.

For instance, there is a higher probability that an individual practising groupwork will by definition know more about how groups function than the group members, in the same way that there is a higher probability that a doctor knows more about illness and injury than his patients. But there is a much lower probability that either the doctor or the groupworker will understand more than the people they work with about the special circumstances of their everyday lives. Thus black people, women, the elderly, the disadvantaged and all others who may be on the point of becoming group members have to make a risk assessment.

Social psychologists are fond of using a cost/reward analysis to describe this kind of situation. But however it is described, what it amounts to is that if the basis of any group is what its members bring into it, and if the success or otherwise of the group is dependent upon how that material is used in the group, then there is a great deal of risk and a high probability of misunderstanding if the potential members cannot be reasonably sure that their particular and different backgrounds and belief systems will at least be known about, and preferably understood.

There are many elements of human situations about which it is possible to know a great deal without actually having experienced them personally. There are others, which are usually of a much more intimate and personal nature, for which it is not. The result of this is that there is often enough a large gap between knowing and understanding, between the individual and the expert in terms of understanding the personal value of that situation.

So if a problem or situation which is to become part of the remit of a group falls into the category of general knowledge, most people will be happy to be dealt with by 'experts', i.e. people who possess that knowledge. But where the problem is one of a social nature, like being a member of an ethnic minority and possibly subject to oppressive and discriminatory attitudes and behaviour, then the perception of being understood is more likely to reside in individuals who have actually experienced that situation for themselves. There are thus some kinds of social experience which can only be truly understood by experiencing them.

The laws of probability give a clear enough reason why large numbers of individuals in society may opt if offered the chance to work with those whose general knowledge is backed by specifically similar experience.

DIFFERENCE AND SIMILARITY

Some differences, as I have just indicated, are almost too great to be understood without personal experience of them; others are exactly what provide the members of a group with ideas and viewpoints about common problems that had not previously occurred to them. It is the diversity of human experience which, if it can be revealed in circumstances where advantage can be taken of its value for learning, provides a considerable amount of the resources which are available to a group. Much will be made of this later.

Many groups, as we have seen, are founded around the fact that their members have some fairly obvious common interest. Indeed, I would go so far as to say that most groups which are created have this as a basic element. But it must be remembered that whatever that common element is, be it drugs, depression, oppression or whatever, the experiences of it that the members will bring to the group, while having common elements, will have more that is idiosyncratic and personal. However, one fact which similarity does have in its favour is that when people with such an element of common experience are brought together, it immediately becomes obvious to all that the aloneness that many have felt in their efforts to cope can be relieved in the perception that others have had similar, albeit not identical, experiences.

In this chapter I have tried to present very briefly the simple fact that groups are composed of individuals whose individuality has been shaped genetically, socially and by reflection on experience. Understanding that this is so is one of the most important steps in enabling the leadership of a group to be able to bring about the sharing, commitment and co-operation of members and leadership which fuels the group. This is the first of the four basic elements of the group process. The second comprises the effects of those factors which are called constraints, both positive and negative, and it is to them we must now turn.

3

SMALL GROUPS AND BIGGER GROUPS

The constraints

Great fleas have little fleas upon their backs
  to bite 'em,
And little fleas have lesser fleas, and so on
  ad infinitum.

Augustus de Morgan,
A Budget of Paradoxes, 1872

No group exists in a social vacuum, no matter how secretive or self-concealing that group may try to be.

Consider. A group comes into existence only because individuals meet, gather together and thus become visible one to another. From that point, if the group continues to exist, each person present starts to place the others as being part of that meeting: the members locate one another in the context of the group because each group as it starts is something which has never existed before exactly in that form with those members.

So it is reasonable to suppose that the conditions under which the group meets, how they are first brought together, their purposes, and many other factors will have some salient effects upon how the group grows and how it manages to function.

In this sense, working with groups is an art of the possible, and an effective groupworker is someone who is able to make a realistic assessment of the possible effects that any given factors which come within the ambit of the proposed group will tend to have upon it. Thus although it may be deemed desirable to attempt to achieve a certain end for a particular group of people, it may not be possible because of the constraints which exist. If this is the case, it may be that the constraints can be altered or allowed for, or the project may have to be reformed in some other way or abandoned altogether. As we shall see, not all constraints are negative in their effects, nor are they necessarily unsupportive. In most cases recognition of their existence is a recognition of a reality, and so aims can be set which are not only beneficial but possible. As I have said, it also needs to be recognized that some constraints can be changed by the application of suitable procedures.

23

Any collection of people therefore which exists as such over a period of time is subject to two major influences: first, the processes which stem from the awareness that each individual has of the presence of others, and consequently of the responses which s/he will tend to produce; and second, all those pressures which arise from the fact that the collection of people does not exist in isolation but is part of larger systems and organizations, and comprises people who belong to other groups as well.

We have seen in Chapter 2 what members of a group bring into that group with them when they become members, and we will see later the major influence those imports have on how the group develops and works, but in this chapter I want to show how factors which are usually seen as external to the group as an entity can and do influence practically every part of it.

No social system is free of the influence of smaller systems which occur within it, nor that of larger ones of which it is a part.

When we look at the characteristics of members of any particular group, we have to remember that those characteristics were acquired outside the current group and that they are very similar, but not identical, to the characteristics of people from the same social system who are not members of the group, and with whom the group members may be in quite frequent contact.

It is rather difficult to distinguish between those influences which group members bring with them into a group and those influences which operate from outside the group's confines. For if we think clearly about it, a lot of those external influences have effect, or apparently so, only because members within the group are aware of them and respond to them. This is not entirely true, as we shall see later. Members may not be wholly aware of some of the factors outside the group and which surround it and to which they are subject. But there is little doubt that lack of awareness of their existence does little to diminish the effects these factors can have. What is very common is that the effect is noticed but wrongly ascribed to some more visible factor operating within the group. For example, a group may meet in a building which is used because it is available but which may be unsuitable – say dingy, or packed with furniture and apparatus used in the room's main functions. This inconvenience may be felt by members to be being overcome by their concentration on their own business, but may nevertheless influence the members and make them unaccountably irritable and frustrated. These feelings will then spill over into their attitudes and behaviour to others in the group, who will then become the focus of blame for the feeling that the group is not working effectively.

Example

A group of teenage probationers was set up by their probation officer to meet on a weekly basis in a room at the local further education college. While in terms of access and availability the college was a good choice, it was unfortunate in that it was unfamiliar to the lads in the group and made them feel very uncomfortable and very conscious of their status of being, as they put it, 'cons'. Their behaviour became defiant, and for some long period of time they were unable to settle down to the tasks of the group.

This was a small example of the effect that environment, in this case a building and its use, can have on the performance of a group. The site had been chosen by the group leader because it was very convenient for all those involved. The amenities were excellent, but the essential fact of its being not only unfamiliar ground to the lads but also a place connected with higher education had not been allowed for in the original plan. It proved unsettling enough to be a large part of the cause of the group's premature ending.

It is not necessary to regard these external influencing factors as always negative. In fact, they are frequently very positive, and indeed when individuals are aware that such influences exist, it is usually possible to use them to assist the group, to allow for them or in some selected cases to remove them or the group to where they will have no effect.

These external factors of influence are often referred to as the 'constraints' under which a group has to operate. Quite frequently they will make the difference between whether a group set up in their ambit will or will not actually work in the way its convenors intended. It is impossible to list all the constraints to which any particular group will be subjected, but I think that if we can manage to define and illustrate even a few, then the basic idea of what to look for and what to expect from them might have been established. I propose that we look at the following rather large examples:

1 the environment in which the group exists;
2 the characteristics and behaviour patterns of its members;
3 the characteristics, behaviour patterns and intentions of group convenors and leaders;
4 the effects of time;
5 the effects of the resources which are available;
6 how the group came into being – its origins;
7 what kind of agreement was made about the group – its contract;
8 the group's task or purpose;
9 the actual size of the group;
10 the nature of the activities the group pursues;
11 whether the group has constant or fluctuating membership.

This may look like a formidable list of possible influences but they are by no means all independently functioning entities and in most cases a brief statement about them should serve to define them and to illustrate their probable sphere of influence. The whole purpose of this exercise is to make group members and leaders, both potential and actual, aware that these factors exist. Quite simply, if we do not know that some elements of a situation exist, then there is no way in which their influences can be taken into our reckoning, with the usual consequence that their effects are ascribed to something entirely erroneous, as we have just seen.

THE ENVIRONMENT

Many groups exist within the confines of a larger organization. By this I mean that even if they do not operate within the premises of that organization, they are set up to fulfil some of its purposes and are therefore subject to its approval and possible funding.

In a more general sense the environment means the actual place where a group operates, the confines of available space, the facilities which are available, its use by other and very different organizations, and its accessibility to those who might wish to become members.

The climate of opinion within an environment is another very important constraint. Groups have been set up in the teeth of hostile opposition which has ultimately proved beneficial because it increased the determination of the group members to succeed, but it can be a very destructive force, particularly if the opposition is not open but covert.

Example

When groups for prisoners were established by the assistant governor of an adult prison most of the prison officers were hostile to the venture, but because the idea had been imposed without real consultation and because the group leaders were professionals from outside the prison staff, no direct opposition to the move was expressed. But when the time came for the groups to assemble for their meetings in different areas of the prison it was always discovered that several prisoners had been already drafted to other duties. As one of the main aims of the groups had been to achieve a stable membership week after week, this ploy completely disrupted the groups and they were eventually abandoned in that particular form.

Alternatively, the manifestation of the environment in the form of its climate can be positively encouraging.

26

Example

A young man who was unemployed lived on a small estate which had become subject to a spate of burglaries. He decided that he would try to do something useful to pass his time productively. He broached the idea of starting a neighbourhood watch scheme, but was informed by his parents and some of his friends that the people living on the estate were too 'enclosed' in the sense of their preferring 'keep themselves to themselves' attitudes rather than being interested in anything that involved co-operative endeavour.

However, when the young man knocked on doors he was pleased to find that the burglaries had changed this traditional attitude quite considerably and he was given a great deal of encouragement – and, more importantly, a large number of individuals volunteered their services. He had no difficulty in recruiting enough people to set up continuous evening patrols through the estate and to help with the organization. The new climate of opinion was a constraint but one which acted positively and encouragingly.

THE CHARACTERISTICS OF THE MEMBERS

As what members bring into a group has been well covered in the previous chapter, it should be reasonably clear how such importations and the resulting behaviour patterns of members can act as quite a major constraint on what a group can achieve. Although a group may well help its members to achieve goals which they had previously thought beyond their reach, this does not alter the fact that all individuals have limitations, which may have been imposed by genetics or by learning or by temperament or by experience and belief. In particular, the way individual members within a group respond and interact with one another will determine to a large extent what they as a group system can achieve. Chief among such personal characteristics which make an essential difference to whether even the simplest, least demanding group actually functions is the element of commitment.

A group – any group – is a small social system which derives its energy and ability to achieve what it was established to do only in the degree that its members will give of their resources of energy, time, skill, knowledge and experience.

Example

A group of neighbours had realized that living in their midst were a elderly couple of whom the wife was seriously ill and confined to bed

27

and wheelchair. Her husband, with the help of carers, was able to look after her. But in so doing he had neither the time, the energy nor the inclination to look after their largish garden, which had once been his wife's great pride. Realizing that she would soon be wanting to go out in her wheelchair to see her garden, the neighbours decided that they would band together as a group and look after it for her. All went well at first as the group worked co-operatively to clear the mess that had developed. But gradually, fewer of the group appeared to be available to do the routine tasks of maintenance until the group had become two people: the immediate neighbours of the old couple and, after them, the people who had lived longest in the area. The garden was still attended to, much to the delight of the old lady, but it was no longer a group enterprise and thus much more limited in scope and much more demanding of the time and commitment of the two who remained.

Of course, there are rules about how people allocate their time and energy to different uses, and one of the simplest is that there has to be some accounting between output and input. Once other available interests become more attractive, then those which are perceived as having greater costs for lesser rewards will tend to be abandoned, especially if the altruism which fuelled the first efforts has to a large extent been dissipated.

This is a constraint which is a constant bugbear to all those who would like to convene or create groups for very specific purposes. Unless a group begins, fairly early in its life, to yield some rewards for the effort of attending and of committing energy and time to it, alternative uses of that energy and time will tend to become much more appealing and members will quit.

THE CHARACTERISTICS, BEHAVIOUR PATTERNS AND INTENTIONS OF GROUP CONVENORS AND LEADERS

It is axiomatic that those who seek to bring a group into existence have some valid (to them) reasons for doing so, and thus it would be only rational to expect that those reasons will have some considerable effect on the eventual form that the group will take. It is also almost always true that convenors of groups have some basic ideas about how the group will be run to achieve the goals that they originally had in mind. Let us look at how these two factors might operate as constraints on a group.

Example

The residents of a small village had over the years come to realize that their main street had become a major through route for large lorries from a big factory which had been established a couple of miles away. Not only were these heavy vehicles noisy, they also created dust in clouds as they drove through, and, more importantly still, they proved dangerous to both the young and the elderly inhabitants, and also to the fabric of the old buildings of the main street. Various individuals had appealed to the local authority to do something, even if only to cause the drivers to slow down when they entered the village precincts, or more effectively to reroute the wagons away from the village altogether. But while vague promises had been made, nothing actually got done. A couple of villagers arranged for a petition to be signed by all, and even this was ignored.

Eventually, one inhabitant convened a village meeting and put forward the idea that they should all unite as a group and that they should block the road continually with their presence until something was done. Many regarded this as an illegal and dangerous exploit, but at last, in desperation, the group organized itself into a systematic series of blockages with signs to warn approaching drivers of the presence of people in the road. The hold-up brought the police, and after a considerable number of fairly acrimonious meetings the village got agreement on the permissible speed of the wagons and negotiations on rerouting, with the reminder that blockages could be restarted any time that they felt they were not getting what they wanted.

The convenor of this village group had clearly had in mind what the group would do and how it would be organized, and despite some reluctance to act in such an aggressive manner on the part of the older and more sedate inhabitants, the group eventually was created and functioned exactly as she had expected. Her idea of the strategy the group would have to pursue had come from reading in a national paper about how a similar impasse had been resolved. But she had also realized some very important facts about group formation which revolve around the idea that it is necessary for someone to see that a problem exists, to believe that they can see some way of resolving it by involving others, and, most important of all, that they feel that they have the ability to do something about it and also that they are prepared to take the risks involved. We will come back to these points again later.

From this example it is possible to see that because there was one person who used her energy, determination and evaluation of the problem to set this group in motion and who kept it going with her encouragement and leadership, the group which emerged was directed by her. Interestingly enough, when the group began to achieve some success, its form and leadership changed from sole director to a committee form as more of the villagers realized that they had something to contribute and that the problems they continued to face did not necessarily need such directive and dynamic leadership.

One final point is that in the more treatment-oriented forms of group, the leaders and convenors frequently subscribe to particular theories of group behaviour and of the most effective group forms to be used. As we will see later, such groups are most clearly defined by these elements of the belief system of the individual leader, even down to the length of time the group meets, the interpretation of the group's behaviour, the admission of members, the duration of sessions, what material is admissible and what not, and so on.

THE EFFECTS OF TIME

In several ways, time is one of the most important of the constraints. For instance, there is the amount of time available for each session, the time between sessions and the length of time for which the group will exist. All these factors should be taken into consideration when a group is being planned. The example given next is taken from a report by a group of social workers on a groupwork project with a group of children.

Example

Social workers were expected to involve themselves in the group in their own leisure time with no lessening of their commitments elsewhere. This meant that the social workers were often tired and lacking in enthusiasm, which can only prevent groups from reaching their full potential . . . other important factors which relate to the success or failure of groupwork are proper communication with parents, schools and other social workers, full discussion of each meeting and written reports. *Time was scarce and for us this meant that all these areas were neglected to some degree and not satisfactorily dealt with.*

In this situation time reduced the possible effectiveness because the amounts of it that were essential to achieve success were not forthcoming. It is a common problem of groupwork that leaders underestimate the amount of time that will need to be available to do the job properly.

Another group from the same project also found that time was an important factor, and the extract from their report given below shows how much time they had to devote to their group.

Example

Wednesday evenings over six months have involved approximately eighty hours' work for each social worker. Added to this are three weekends and one Sunday as well as many hours, mainly within normal working time spent discussing the group and planning. Without taking the weekends into consideration this represents a conservative estimate of a 10 per cent increase on each social worker's workload.

THE NATURE OF THE AVAILABLE RESOURCES.

I have already hinted that people are an important constraint. Indeed they are, but they are also the main resource any group possesses, as we shall examine in some detail later. But first let me give an example of what can happen when other resources are not made available in an appropriate way.

Example

Some years ago a group of social workers in a large city area had decided that they would attempt to establish a group for children on the basis that it would form an intermediate treatment group. Now the concept of such a group, while partly accepted by their authority, had at that time never before been put into practice. When the authority was asked to give its blessing to the project, it hedged all its bets. The group could proceed but only on the condition (a) that it did not cost the authority anything, (b) that it was not held during the time when the social workers were legally employed by the authority, (c) that it was clearly recognized that there was no official underpinning for the project, (d) that there would be no requests for reduced workloads in order to have time to work with the project and so on . . .

What might have had endless possibilities, given minimal backing by the authority, was hamstrung by lack of resources, tiredness on the part of the staff, and suspiciousness on the part of other agencies at the apparent lack of official support. The effectiveness of the project would have been dependent largely upon the energy and goodwill of those involved, who incidentally were not given any help by those who had already gone through the experience of setting up just such a group and whose expertise could have saved them a lot of time and trouble.

THE ORIGINS OF GROUPS

At the risk of over-simplifying the matter, I would say that there are at least five main situations from which groups might arise:

1 The group is already in existence.
2 It just happened.
3 It arose from public or partially public advertisement.
4 It arose from a large public meeting which split into smaller group units.
5 It was created by individual selection from a known public.

This list makes plain a fact, often ignored by groupworkers, that created groups are not necessarily the closed, intense-experience units which so often seem to be regarded as the norm. Such groups are only one end of a fairly large continuum, at the other end of which are large communities comprising many not too clearly defined smaller groups.

One other fact needs to be made clear also, which is that the way a group originates acts as a constraint on that group and tends to dominate its life from start to finish.

Groups already in existence

Prime examples of groups already in existence are those which are usually considered to be 'natural', e.g. the family, the gang, the work group, the friendship group. We will consider this definition of some groups as 'natural' in some detail later. The main identifying feature of all these groups is that they were set up to meet certain human needs and this causes their members to have a particular idea about the group and their membership of it. For instance, few families have ever thought of themselves as a 'group' in quite the sense that a family groupworker might do when exposing the 'dynamics' of the group. They will customarily have thought of themselves as family members, part of their kith and kin with specifically defined relationships to each other.

Likewise, a groupworker may take over a street gang, each member of which has a view of his place in that gang, and will try to engage them in seeing other kinds of relationships within it that, while unfamiliar, no doubt exist.

Groups that just happen

A group that 'just happened' is much the same as the first category, but instead of someone from outside the group coming to shove it into seeing itself as a different kind of group, in this case it is usually done by some member of the group.

There are many examples of the way that a group seems to emerge spontaneously to meet an arising situation. What usually happens is that individuals have a perception of the situation and make moves to start actions which they see as necessary to meet it, and in so doing they pull others along with them. When a group forms in this way its structure and performance and the commitment of its members are all largely dependent on the way it grew.

Groups arising from advertisement or selection

Groups which arise from public advertisement or from a public meeting are likewise dominated during their life, at least in the early stages, by virtue of the way in which they were created.

Those groups which are created by selection are inevitably marked by the process of their creation, for selection usually means not only that those who are chosen have been selected on the basis of some idea by the convenor, but also that they all tend to have something of importance in common. For instance, a groupworker may choose as members of his/her group known clients with a similar problem. The exclusivity of this approach, while producing some very important benefits, as we shall see later, also has the effect of defining to a large extent how the group will function. The very nature of the choice of members limits and constrains the group.

THE NATURE OF ANY AGREEMENT ABOUT THE GROUP

If a contract can be defined as a working agreement between a group leader or convenor and the prospective members of a group, then that contract will define to quite a considerable extent how the group will function. Although contracts can be renegotiated as the group grows and changes, it will have been set upon its way by the initial agreement as much as it would by the process of selection. (More on this in Chapter 7.)

THE GROUP'S TASK OR PURPOSE

The constraint operating to restrict the group's task or purpose is the simple fact that if the group chooses to do one thing, then it is automatically prevented from doing something else at the same time.

THE SIZE OF THE GROUP

The size of a group – that is, the number of members it has – obviously must have some effect on the way it works. Take a very simple example: if a group has a given period of time in which to comĕ to a particuar decision, then the amount of time which can be allocated to each member to get ideas across is a function of three things: the organization of the group; the forcefulness or otherwise of individual members; and time. The last of these is important because if all members are to contribute their thinking to the debate and there are many members, then the amount of time each can be allowed is small. If some members are more forceful than others they may hog what time is available and in so doing deprive less pushy members of the time to have their say.

If a group has many members, there is the possibility of more ideas being produced, but equally there is the chance that for at least some of the membership there will be little time in which to express them unless some powerful element of control is exercised by leaders or the group itself.

Conversely, if a group is small there may be fewer ideas available but it will be more likely that there will be sufficient time for them to be expressed.

These are obviously general ideas because what is small in one context may be large in another. But usually when intensity of personal contact is an important part of the group's remit, low numbers are essential, based on roughly how many people it is possible to contact on a face-to-face basis. Where the activity of the group is general and social, a group can be quite large because it will tend to split into smaller ones. (Subgroups will be dealt with later.)

Practical facts arising from the effect of numbers are few. However, odd numbers will favour the reaching of a decision in voting behaviour. Also, large groups provide the probability that some members will be able to avoid taking any active part in proceedings and, as has been said, small groups generally intensify the personal contacts between members. Large groups usually have more of a problem of communication unless there is some kind of structure which facilitates it. It is also much easier for members of large groups to come and go without affecting the group's business or its culture too much.

THE ACTIVITIES THE GROUP CHOOSES
TO PURSUE

All groups pursue activities of some kind, and it is manifestly obvious that what those actitivities are will constrain some aspects of the kind of group that emerges. There is a somewhat tricky point involved here, for in many instances created groups are set up to achieve given purposes, and then the activities which the group will pursue are decided on the basis of how best to achieve those purposes. Yet by choosing some activities rather than others in the pursuit of the group's aims, the future shape of the group and its processes have largely been determined, at least until some new change of activity takes place. Thus a group which chooses to confront its members' problems by a combination of role play and discussion will develop differently from one which chooses to deal with similar problems by a process of information-giving.

THE EFFECTS OF A CONSTANT OR FLUCTUATING MEMBERSHIP

Groups which never close their doors to the admission of acceptable new members, like social clubs, are usually called 'open' groups, and the effects of fluctuating membership are usually clearly visible. Such groups never seem to develop the intense personal relationships across the whole group; they do have some difficulties in maintaining a sufficient number of core members to transmit the group culture.

The alternative type of group which is defined as 'closed' has a supposedly constant membership, with the result that it acts on a more intense level with fewer relationships and does not have the problem of initiating new members or of the transmission of culture. It does, however, lack the possible stimulus of new members and consequently has a higher risk of stagnation.

There have been several hints during this chapter that the constraints we have been considering are not always immovable. Indeed, some groups have been established in order to change constraints which affected the functioning of their members. The effects of the characteristics of members can, for instance, be radically changed by introducing new members to a group who are known or thought to have the skills and behaviours which the group, as originally constituted, apparently lacks. Resources might possibly be added to or changed, and leaders' attitudes and ideas influenced into different and more appropriate channels. The time available can be discussed and maybe reallocated or extended or changed in other ways. Contacts can be renegotiated as circumstances within the group can be seen to have changed. Even the tasks and purposes of the group can be varied as it becomes aware of the fact that this might be expedient or necessary. The structure of the group can be modified, its activities reviewed and changed accordingly, and its size and the freedom of access of new members to it altered as required.

Very few of the constraints I have listed here are wholly immovable. The basic requirements for dealing with constraints are simple. First, realize that they exist; second, realize their likely effects; and third, work out how best they can be set aside or more effectively used as positive rather than as negative influences.

The third of the four basic elements of group process which we must consider next comprises the effects of combining the other three. That is, it consists of the processes which develop when group members, constraints and leadership acts operate within the confined social space of a small group.

4

WHAT HAPPENS IN GROUPS
Group processes

To reiterate, the absolutely basic form of any group is that a number of people gather together in a given place for a period of time. When people gather together in this way where they can see one another and become aware of each other's presence, their behaviour most usually tends to begin to take account of those presences. In simple language, each individual's behaviour is subtly modified by that individual's being aware of coming under the scrutiny of others. How those modifications of behaviour emerge and the forms they take become the basic characteristics of any group.

Furthermore, what kind of behaviour will actually emerge depends to a great extent on each group member's previous experience of similar situations. This means that the whole of the relevant experience of which the individual is more or less aware will be brought into play in order that some degree of safety can be assured. For, as we have seen, the fear, the basic fear of being forced into a position of having to regard oneself as isolated, rejected and alone, is sufficient to make most of us try very hard to be accepted and thus reduce a strange, new situation to something which is less strange and threatening and more comfortable to live with.

The acts of leadership, which we will consider in some detail later, are in fact a special case of the process I have just described – special because most leaders have that position because they have learned, in addition to the learning they acquired during their growing-up period, to recognize how the interaction of people in group situations tends to proceed and to observe how in any particular group the processes are shaping, with what intensity and to what ends. They have also learned how these processes are generated by the ideas and experience and desires of the people who comprise the membership of any group and the ways in which influence to change or modify that generation, if it should be deemed necessary, can be brought about.

Thus all groups produce what can be called 'processes'. All that this word means is that there are discernible patterns of behaviour which tend to emerge in groups over time and appear to focus around certain aspects of the group's behaviour – for example, around the relationships that develop, or around the rule and value systems to which it adheres. It is possible to see these patterns developing and it is possible to influence their development in various ways and to various ends. They arise quite simply from the fact that people bring into a group with them ideas, beliefs, energy, attitudes, needs and desires, and a whole bundle of behavioural patterns from their past experience, aptitudes and abilities, skills and problems; in fact, their whole being.

In the confined social space in which a group operates, with some of the constraints described in the previous chapter in place, the group behaviour patterns which we describe as 'processes' emerge. In this chapter we are going to look at how this occurs, what effects the emergence has, what values for the group they have and how they can be influenced and to what ends.

Wherever a collection of people exists as such over a period of time, inevitably certain things will occur, if only a recognition of the fact that the collection exists and that each individual sees him/herself in some discrete way as belonging to it. In a way this recognition does not even require a basic commitment on the part of the individual except to be there with all the others. It does not even require his/her willingness to be there, though there is a much greater chance of what has been called a 'formed' group developing if his/her physical presence *is* accompanied by a degree of commitment to that collection of individuals.

The processes which have been most commonly recognized by groupworkers and theorists as arising are as follows:

The most fundamental process of all:	Interaction
The structural processes:	Group development
	Roles and status
	Subgroup formation
The operational processes:	Goal formation
	Decision-making
	Using resources
The regulating processes:	Setting norms, standards and values
	Developing cohesion
	Acquiring influence
	Developing an ethos

THE FUNDAMENTAL PROCESS: INTERACTION

'Interaction' is a word used by psychologists and others to describe in one general term the very complex business of the way in which people actively engage in responding to the presence of others. Frequently, interaction has been limited to meaning only the visible verbal and gestural response patterns. But in reality it should be held to cover also the thought processes and feelings which are not necessarily expressed in the form of speech or action. The social intercourse which takes place between members of a group is what eventually generates most of the processes by which the group will operate.

When individuals are aware that there are others in their presence, especially when those others have been gathered together for some purpose common to all, they tend to react to these presences in a variety of habitual ways. If an attempt to ignore the presence of others is the response, then it must be understood that it is essential to know that others exist before they can be ignored.

Depending on how we feel towards others in our space, so reactions will be tempered. The degree of our need to be accepted by others will be a great factor in the kind of attitudes and behaviour we display.

If we take a group of people who are brought together because they are facing a common problem, whatever that might be, then before they can begin to operate as a group – that is, as an integrated unit – a whole large area of security needs to be cleared up. During the course of talking, observing and acting together, the members of a group like this will begin to use established ways of assuring themselves that what they entered into is going to have some rewards for them. They are going to form impressions about the other members of the group and whatever leaders there happen to be, and they are going to have feelings ranging from liking to disliking, from wanting to stay to wanting to get out, from suspicion to the beginnings of trust. They are going to try to establish in their own ways what their position in the group is liable to be in relation to the position of others and whether it is one which will carry sufficient reward to be worth the risks which may be involved.

All this and much more occurs because the individuals involved will interact with one another, they will communicate with each other, they will weigh one another on the scales of past experience and they will make judgements.

One reason for bringing together a group of people who have a common problem is very simply that they will all have tried in various ways to find a solution or way of coping with it. Some will have been more successful than others and some may have been totally defeated by the problem. If it now becomes possible for the individuals in the group to share their experiences in the ways in which they coped or did not cope, then each stands a chance of learning something new which may be of value and help in their own coping.

Often enough, people can do this grouping of resources for themselves except for one important fact, which is that they are frequently unaware that there may be other people in the same boat as themselves or of where they may contact them. There is also the fact that they may be afraid of the reception they might receive if they tried. Given that sharing experience can increase by a considerable margin the resources of coping which become available, a group can create the kind of situation where the essential inter-action can lead to a level of trust developing which is appropriate for that kind of exchange to take place.

Interaction is the basic common process of all groups. Everything else which occurs in the group arises from the interaction of its members – not just in the quantity of the interaction but very much also in its quality and what value it has for the individual members.

THE STRUCTURAL PROCESSES

Group development

A somewhat confusing state of affairs exists in the literature on groupwork about the idea of group development, largely because 'development' is dynamic and can be regarded as a 'process', and is therefore attributed to a group as one of its integral characteristics. Thus when some texts use the word 'process', the writers intend it to stand for the way in which a group appears to grow and change over the course of its existence. This is based upon the idea that a group can be considered as an entity in its own right, whereas a more common-sense approach would be content to say that what changes are the behavioural patterns of the individual members as they grow more at home with being in the group and working with others.

Nevertheless, groups do change over time, if only due to a process of famil-iarization and the development of the ability to predict what fellow members are liable to do. Thus changes in the group's overall behavioural patterns occur as members interact with one another. New experiences, different moods, perceptions and understandings, learning and support arise as the group continues to meet.

If interchange does not take place, the group either disintegrates or stag-nates. Stagnation is sometimes found in groups in residential homes for elderly people, where little or no stimulation from outside occurs and the group itself generates none. Residents can become apathetic and routine bound, where the most important event of any day is a meal-time. If this goes on for a long time, they will come to lose any ability to change and will in fact often resent change when it is offered because of the effort which will be needed to achieve it.

The fact that all groups change when they have stimulation is one thing; to say that they develop is another and different thing. Development implies that there is some perceptible order or direction about the change, and this is pre-cisely what group theorists imply when they talk about the developmental stages of a group. Development can be likened to the maturation process of a child who gradually learns about him/herself and his/her abilities and about the surrounding environment, including important adults. But even this is not a totally accurate picture. A group develops because it is a social unit comprising separate individuals who have the ability to recognize more or less clearly that in order to achieve whatever ends the group was created for, they will need to come to terms with individual differences and learn to co-operate at an appropriate level.

Development in a group tends to imply that all groups which survive, or at least those that do not stagnate, appear to move towards a more efficient use of their resources. Many people have attempted to define what this development looks like, and most seem to be content to say that it occurs in definable stages. What is clear is that if an observer were to examine a group at work at different times during its existence, s/he would invariably find that there were marked changes in the way in which the group operated. Indeed, there are well-marked points which occur in the life of any group, but they are not necessarily progressive in the sense that stage 2 always appears after stage 1 and so on. Nor is it any more accurate to replace this linear sequence with one that is partly regressive. Experience tends to show that:

1 Some groups hardly ever show any kind of change. Maybe it is not necessary that they should change in order to achieve their purpose, maybe it is not within the group's ability to do so. There may be many reasons, both internal and external.

   (a) Some people in a group see and feel the need to change before others and bring pressure to bear on them to follow suit. This sometimes results in individuals who may appear to be holding the group back being subjected to quite strong aggression, which causes attention and energy that should have been devoted to the group's business to be used in non-productive ways. If the problem of different speeds amongst the members is resolved, then the group may be free to pursue its progress.

   (b) Some groups seem to fluctuate in that they make progress and then regress and seem to need to go back over some of the ground they have already covered in order to consolidate it. This often occurs when a group has moved too fast and is uncertain of its current position and needs to go back to a position of safety and rebuild slowly.

   (c) Some areas of group behaviour develop more quickly and soundly than others. For instance, a group of strangers can sometimes discover something that they all have in common (beyond their common humanity, that is), which can very quickly develop a sense of being in the same boat. The actual understanding of each other as people may in no way have kept pace with this emotional warmth generated by the perceived similarity, and it is sometimes very easily demonstrated to be a false dawn when the group is subjected to pressure commensurate with its apparent level of development.

2   Different stages in the life of a group allow it to cope with different kinds of stress. The point is illustrated by the difference between a group which is just a collection of people and one which has been in existence long enough for it to be aware of its potential and to be able to work together as a unit, using its resources. In the early stages of a group's progress it is composed of individuals whose prime motivation is often to ensure their personal safety in a relatively unknown situation, and the pursuit of the group's business, whatever that might be, is often a poor second.

This can mean that the sort of pressure which a group can tolerate may well be related to the stage of its development. This is a point of crucial interest, for many groups have been asked to perform tasks that require a level of co-operation from the members which they are wholly unprepared to give because they have not become sufficiently integrated into the group, or experienced what level of support it is able to give them. Incidentally, when a task can be performed by individual members of the group rather than by the group acting as a whole, unless what they do is integrated into the group pattern there is a very real danger that such behaviour will begin to create gaps in the fabric of the group. There are many so-called groups in which there are doers and hangers-on or watchers, which tends to create two subgroups with very different levels of satisfaction in their membership.

The end point of the development of a group is when it has achieved what it set out to do or when it is forced to realize that such an end is indeed impossible. Some groups of course do not end; they are open and the membership is continually changing, and their development is much flatter and slower than that of small, closed groups which do stop when they have achieved their end point.

One final word about group development. Where groups have leaders and members who are aware that groups are supposed to have a developmental sequence, there is a much greater probability that such a sequence will actually emerge.

Consider: the group processes are patterns which emerge from the interaction between various elements – that is, the characteristics of the members; the constraints under which the group operates; the tasks which it sets itself to perform; and the element of direction which it receives from any leaders it may have. Given that group leaders tend to have more experience of how groups operate than their members, the degree of influence that they can exert over how the group develops is considerable and probably more than they are consciously aware of. As they have very probably learned that groups

41

are expected to develop, it would be very surprising if they did not. In any case, a very large part of a groupworker's skill will certainly reside in helping a group produce the level of development compatible with its being able to achieve its defined ends.

Roles and status

During the course of a group's existence, certain members will own up to having, and will often demonstrate, abilities of various kinds. Where these abilities appear to be of value to the group in the pursuit of its aims, these members may be asked, and will often agree, to do particular jobs. If these jobs become an acceptable part of the group's behaviour, then the process of creating a role structure within the group is in being. For instance, there may be one person in the group who always seems to be the one to whom other members turn for advice, or there may be one who can always be relied upon to remind others that time is running out and they need to get on with the task in hand.

A structure is created by virtue of the expectation of members that certain roles will be fulfilled. That is, certain roles become identified with certain members because they have been seen to perform these roles frequently enough for it to become predictable. When this happens, the group has a social structure which can be recognized not only by those within the group who have seen it grow but by any reasonably percipient observer from outside the group. Some roles relate to the power the individual role performers have in being able to influence the way the group functions. Thus certain members are seen as possessing enhanced status, which in effect means that they appear to other members to possess abilities and attributes which other members admire or which are seen as being of value to the group as a whole. Often status is related to an individual's experience, usually of the kind which elicits a form of admiration or envy in others. Some high-status members possess personalities which are dominant and forceful, and are seen as able to protect those they accept as followers. In short, many factors contribute not just to a structure of expected performance roles but also to a hierarchy or ranking amongst the members.

Subgroup formation

It is a ubiquitous fact of group life that large groups contain smaller groupings within their boundaries, and larger groups are usually part of even larger groups or organizations. Within the small groups which groupworkers set up, smaller groups form and re-form as need and interest vary. Some become permanent features. Others are transient, brought into being by a current need. Once that need is met, the group disintegrates and other, more appropriate subgroups are formed.

Members tend to cluster around those others whom they like or who appear to be powerful enough to ensure that personal ends can be achieved; alliances are developed in order that pressure can be brought to bear in the group to achieve desired ends, and some subgroups are formed because of past knowledge of each other or because liking for one another has developed.

In the course of working together, members of a group will discover affinities with other members and so will tend to band together for support. Subgroups will form around people or ideas, and provided they are not too opposed to the mainstream objectives of the whole group, it is from such groups that most of the new ideas and the inspirations tend to come. This is not to say that an individual with good ideas cannot also influence the group as well, but unless s/he is a very strong or very respected (high-status) member of the group, s/he will usually seek support for his/her ideas from others, and then a subgroup will be in the process of being created. Subgroups also form a possible base for members wishing to rebel or to opt out, because they can form a support system capable of making some members feel strong enough to challenge the system as it currently exists.

THE OPERATIONAL PROCESSES

Goal formation

Most, if not all, groups have a purpose, more or less recognized by their members, as the reason for their existence. Whatever the main reason for the group's creation, during the course of its existence other ends will no doubt come into focus and need to be built into the group's programme in an acceptable way. There are several ways in which changes and additions and deletions to the group's agenda can be made, but one fact has emerged innumerable times from all aspects of the study of groups, which is that where the members of a group take an active part in deciding where the group is going and how it will proceed, there is considerably more commitment to that programme by those members than to any programmes generated in any other way.

The goals, aims or purposes of a group may be many and varied. They may comprise goals which individual members of the group find important for themselves; there may be goals which the organizers and supporters of the group have in mind for it; there may be goals which members have in mind for the whole group; and there may be goals which are immediate and those which are long term. If a degree of chaos exists about all these sources of goals, then the group will soon cease to exist as a group and nothing will have been achieved except disappointment. Thus part of the early work of any collection of people hoping to become a group must be to try to sort out what kind of aims each member has for him/herself and for the group as a whole.

This is easier said than done, for two very simple reasons. First, most people entering a group tend to believe that their understanding of the group's purpose is roughly the same as everyone else's. It isn't. However the group was formed, each potential member will have put an idiosyncratic interpretation upon the information received about it, though there will certainly be common elements. Second, whatever personal ends the members may have, they may not – at least in the early stages of a group – wish to have these ideas exposed.

Decision-making

All groups which survive make decisions about what they exist to do and about how it can be achieved. In some cases these decisions are made by individuals who for one reason or another are strong or who feel that they are more aware of what is needed. But even when this occurs there is still a need to carry the rest of the group, or at least some significant part of it, along with the decision. Each group has the potential to develop its own decision-making process. In order to maintain the satisfaction of members with their membership at as high a level as possible, they need to feel that they have some say in what the group is doing. Nothing causes members of any organization to feel completely powerless more quickly than for them to realize that they have no chance of even being involved in the decision-making processes which will substantially affect their lives.

Decisions are made about procedure, about the rules of behaviour, about organization, admission to the group and about expulsion from it, and about the multitude of details of the daily running of the group. But unless what eventually evolves and is clearly seen by the members to exist is a well-defined process of decision-making to which all have equal access, then some members will feel that this process diminishes them and any attraction the group might have had for them.

Using resources

Learning to use the resources within the group, and any outside resources to which it may have access, is perhaps one of the most important processes which occur. The use of material resources is perhaps obvious: things like equipment, films, video, television, toys, books, furniture, buildings and of course money. But the far more important assets are those human resources which are available or potentially available for the group to use. The principal problem in using human resources is, first, discovering that they exist, for many who come into groups believe that they are there because either they have no resources or they have the wrong ones, or that what they have has been of little use. As I hope to show later, this is where the differences between members can be a source of inspiration and hope, disclosing ways of coping which have never previously been thought of. Moreover, there is the support, a very important human resource, which others who really understand from personal experience can offer.

THE REGULATING PROCESSES

Setting norms, standards and values

In order for a collection of individuals to be able to achieve a level of appreciation of themselves and of others within their group which will allow them to share and exchange, to support and criticize, to disclose and be open, to receive and give information and feelings, the processes have to be regulated in some way. As we have seen, when individuals become group members they bring with them the habitual response patterns which they have learned in the course of their lives, in whatever area of society it may be. For instance, they may have learned that nobody ever listens to what they have to say unless they are belligerent and use violent gestures. Most groups founded by group-workers will offer standards of acceptable behaviour for group members in the form of a limited but very important set of rules. For instance, they will usually be very concerned to establish a degree of respect for all members. Probably they will insist on banning violent or racist behaviour, and will lay down some simple rules of procedure, as for instance that everyone has an equal right to be heard.

However, these initial standards tend to be modified as the group continues to exist, and the members and the leaders work on establishing particular rules which fit the members and what the group is trying to achieve. In other words the initial norms and standards are part of a pump-priming exercise which tends to stop the group tearing itself apart in its early stages, until it can become stable enough to discuss and agree its own standards.

Often there may have been no conscious decision about behaviours which are or are not acceptable. But nevertheless, commonly agreed norms establish themselves by virtue of members seeing what happens, what works and what doesn't. Individuals will produce behaviour which apparently transgresses the unwritten standards of behaviour and will be subjected to expressions of disapproval ranging from outright confrontation to a more subtle withdrawal of acceptance of the offending person.

Developing cohesion

Over a period of time, group members may come to feel a kind of emotional bond for their fellow members. It tends to be based upon having shared a considerable number of experiences with them in the confines of the group. This bond tends to divide those who are members of the group from those who are not. Group membership is an exclusive activity just as much as it is inclusive.

Group bonding shows as a feeling of attraction that members have to their group and is usually marked by the amount of time and energy they are prepared to commit to it rather than spend on other activities. The usual term to describe this process is that of developing cohesion.

Groupwork literature has in the past tended to over-emphasize the value of this process. Granted, it is very important, but it has negative aspects, as for instance when a group becomes so cohesive that it stagnates, as no outside influence or breath of fresh air can penetrate its exclusive boundaries. There is also the fact to consider that a large number of groups do not need a very high level of cohesion to perform their functions; a mere agreement to co-operate is all that is required. There is also the possibility that a very cohesive group can maintain bad ideas and standards with exactly the same fervour as we can expect that other groups will generate good ones.

Acquiring influence

Groups are effective in supporting and in changing the behaviour of their individual members because a group can exert pressure. This is an extension of the need for acceptance mentioned earlier. If an individual believes that a group can provide some rewards for him/her, then that group can exert a pressure to conform to its requirements for that individual up to, but not beyond, the point where some other way of achieving his/her ends becomes more acceptable. Obviously if a group holds little interest for a member, then if the pressure to do what the group wishes that member to do becomes too great, he/she will cut his/her losses and leave. If this is not possible, as with groups in prison or with treatment groups that carry penalties for withdrawal, then the member's leaving will take the form either of psychological withdrawal or of sabotaging the group.

It is essential that groups recognize and learn how to handle the process of influence and power, for it is the most potent element both in changing and supporting acceptable levels of behaviour and of overcoming the powerlessness to which many in our society feel themselves subjected.

Developing an ethos

Groups develop what can be described as a 'climate' – an atmosphere which is recognizable in the same way that the characteristics of an individual are recognizable. Individuals who have been in many groups can quite clearly describe the different climates which have obtained in their various groups. Some are friendly, some are deadly serious; some work hard, others seem to get just as much done with an atmosphere of lightheartedness and fun as the main climate, and so on. Others are sullen and resentful because the members are not there because they wish to be. Of course, what the group is doing may well have a great deal of bearing on what kind of ethos is engendered, but this

46

is not the sole cause. Groups, if they are effective, tend to develop the kind of climate which is conducive to their completing the task they have in hand. It is noticeable that groups which are markedly ineffective, tend to have climates which fluctuate wildly and which tend to express the elements of chaos that exist within the group.

Most of these 'processes' are not wholly independent of the others. Indeed, it would be truer to say that each as it develops within a group tends to affect the development of the others. Nor do they all always occur in all groups, but as long as the society from which group members come demonstrates the development of certain belief systems in preference to others, then so will those beliefs become the foundation of the processes which appear in small groups. By making those processes highly visible and by demonstrating their consequences within the group, there arises the possibility that some of the behaviour patterns can be converted in various ways. It is how the processes develop and can be used which is the subject of Part II of this book. But first we must look at the fourth basic element, which is the effects of leadership in its different forms.

5

GUIDANCE, ENABLING
AND DIRECTION

Leadership acts

This chapter draws together most of the more essential ideas about leadership, but as the book as a whole is about working with groups, it is inevitable that ideas about specific aspects of leadership can be found scattered throughout its chapters in appropriate places.

Perhaps one of the most written about and yet most controversial areas of group behaviour concerns those acts which are intentional and directed at influencing the group outcome. Such acts cover the whole concept of leadership and leadership acts and are of great importance in all groups, but more particularly in those which are created to meet specific needs and to achieve particular aims. In current Western society there has developed a degree of suspicion of leadership which is equated with authoritarianism and with people who can be regarded as 'specialists'. Thus, the concept of direction in groups is one of extremely topical interest.

THE NATURE OF LEADERS AND
LEADERSHIP ACTS

Traditionally, leaders have been seen as those who appear to possess specific characteristics such as the ability to influence the behaviour of others; or the ability to command respect for their judgement or acumen; or who just have some natural gift which will allow them to take control of situations that other people have been unable to control.

It is no accident that over the years I must have been asked more questions about how leadership acts are performed than on any other groupwork topic. It is simply that people who set up groups want to know what are the best ways in which their creations can achieve their objectives, and equally those who join groups as members want to know what kind of guidance or directions those who make leadership acts will need to exercise in order for the group to be successful.

One of the more obvious facts about good leaders is that they usually turn

48

out to have received an adequate training in the appropriate skills. As I hope to show later, a fundamental skill is to be able to observe people in a group and note what is going on – that is, to be able to see where the current behaviour in the group is heading and whether it is where the group actually wants or needs to go. Let me settle one point of controversy about leaders straight away, which is that there are all kinds of leader strategies and that one is not necessarily always better than another. Leadership strategies are comparable to a bag of tools: some are more applicable to certain situations than others and, when rightly and appropriately used, just as effective. And also, such strategies can come in certain group conditions just as effectively from those who are designated 'members' as from those designated 'leaders'.

A leader in the first instance is a person who has been given that role by the organization for which s/he works and whose job it is probably to form the group and afterwards to attempt to guide it in the way s/he sees as being important for it to go.

In Chapter 3 on constraints we looked at the ways in which groups originate. In nearly every case the initiative in starting a group came from one or more persons who believed that to start and run a group would be a good way of meeting a particular situation. The implication behind this is simple and it is often one of the first acts of a leader – that is, to see that some form of group may actually be the best way to tackle the problems and needs exposed in certain situations. In the literature this is often referred to as the act of conceptualization. Those who are good at conceptualizing the need for a group are not necessarily equally good at the leadership jobs which immediately follow if the concept is turned into action.

There are discernible points in the range of leader behaviour as listed below. Few exist in entirely pure form, so they are usually found as a dominant or preferred mode. We will look at each in turn.

CONCEPTUALIZATION

We have discussed at length how groups work and the processes which are involved. The act of conceptualization is one of deciding how best, if at all, to set up a group which will make best use of those processes in achieving some defined goals. There are many examples of this kind of preparatory thinking in the groupwork literature so I will quote only one or two here as examples.

Example

The Coventry City Centre Project some years ago identified groups of young people who moved within the rather nebulous, provincial, drug subculture and either misused drugs or were 'at risk'. Having done this,

49

the workers decided that some form of self-help group would be appropriate to this situation. What they actually came up with was a 'self-regulating co-operative' of young people who were involved in identifying ways of helping each other with problems.

In some rural areas children frequently do not have the chance to meet one another, and their parents likewise. Playgroups could be conceptualized as a way to alleviate this difficulty, and when established in this kind of community would provide a point of contact, offering a chance to both groups to meet and socialize.

Individuals being discharged from psychiatric units may need some kind of support to enable them to adapt to life in the community or at least give them a location to which they could go to meet social workers and other individuals in a situation similar to their own for support, help, advice and a stable spot in an otherwise probably uncaring milieu.

A great deal of thinking has to be gone through before any moves are actually made to start a group. At least, that is so in general, but there are occasions when a group is deemed to be essential to deal with a crisis situation which will not give time for a thorough consideration of how best it should be formed. Then the process of conceptualization is short in order to get some form of collective off the ground. How it develops, what form it takes, instead of being a separate and pre-formation activity becomes part of the group's work. This sort of beginning often occurs in groups which are established to meet community issues that threaten a local area with a time scale which has been pre-set by, say, developers or the local authority. An example would be the proposed closure of a small local school without due consultation with those for whom it is an essential institution.

The easiest way to approach the setting up of a group is to ask a series of pertinent questions to which the answers should be at least fairly clear. The first of these questions is undoubtedly, 'Why do I want to set up this group?' The answer may vary from 'Because I am excited about the idea of running a group' to a very clear statement on the lines of 'I want to run this group because I think I can see that there exist a number of individuals who have at least one need which I think can be met most effectively by bringing them together so that they can share their experience of, say, their common problem or their need for support or information'.

The second statement can only be truly made by someone who has a good idea of what a group has to offer. But sharing experiences is a very common reason for starting a group. Many people believe that their particular problem is unique to them, and they not infrequently derive a great deal of encouragement and support when they find themselves in a situation where they have a chance to realize that this is not true and that they are far from being alone with their problem. Whether this occurs or not, there is always the fact that when people have tackled a problem in isolation they have used the resources which they had available to them. These are very seldom the same for everyone, and the fact that they can be shared means that some individuals in the group will be exposed to ways of tackling their problem which had just never occurred to them before.

Some such ideas of sharing form the basis of many very successful groups, and when this occurs it has the added force that when individuals have been in the same boat as one another they are much more likely to accept each other's experience as genuine, a different kind of knowledge from that of the theoretical expert.

Many other questions need to be asked at this thinking stage, especially along the lines of 'Is it possible?', which is the question about resources, both material and in terms of skill. It is also about whether the time is available, whether the agency for which one works is really going to allow a group approach to its clients, and so on. Colleagues have to be consulted, as their goodwill is absolutely necessary if the group is to get off the ground. They don't have to be wildly enthusiastic about the project, just tolerant enough to give it breathing space to prove itself. All these factors we have already come across under the heading of 'constraints', and they will constantly recur during our consideration of working with individuals in groups. This is largely because a poor consideration of these constraints and the ways in which they can affect group outcomes is one of the main causes of the failure of a group.

It should be made clear at this stage that I am not advocating that the constraints which are deemed to exist in any given situation should be regarded as immovable and never looked at in terms of possible change. Indeed, some groups are set up with such change as the very reason for their existence. But it should always be recognized that there are some constraints which will prove to be unchangeable, and the effects these can have on the group should be allowed for where possible in the planning at this stage. It may well emerge that having regard to what constraints exist, the operational aims of the group will have to be modified as the original concept will clearly not be capable of achievement.

ORGANIZATION

Perhaps the first and most important part of organizing a group is to consider its design. The idea of 'designing' a group may sound rather false to many on the grounds that, while a house or a car is an inanimate object and therefore subject to the planning process, such applied to human beings has a ring of artificiality about it. But let us for a moment consider the alternatives. If no planning is involved, then anyone can gather together a haphazard collection of people with no real idea of what they or anyone else wants to do; no goals would have been set and no methods of doing anything would have been established. Whatever the problems of such a collection of people, they would hardly be improved or even revealed by this kind of approach.

However, if such a collection were started and there was a bit of basic planning behind it – for example, if it were decided that the collection would try to mill around and get to know one another slightly and then sit down and try to sort out by a discussion what resources they might have between them which could then be used to help the less fortunate members – then a very different picture might emerge.

Basically, the design of any group must be essentially concerned with its purpose. Once it has been decided to set up a group to meet some kind of situation, then all the factors which will help or hinder that group in achieving its operational end of dealing with that situation have to be considered. Some will certainly be seen to be potentially more beneficial than others and they will need to be given priority in the planning.

For instance, if it is felt that the best way of introducing people to the problems of adoption is to get a group of parents interested in adoption to meet together with some parents who have already adopted children, and ask them to share their ideas, feelings and experience of adoption, then certain factors assume greater importance than others. It becomes necessary to have a meeting room in which the invitees can not only feel relaxed but also move about fairly freely and talk to one another in a manner to which they are all accustomed and under no pressure. The number of meetings will need to be small, probably dictated by the operational aim of the group, which is the exchange of information, feelings and experience, and under relaxed circumstances this should not take a great deal of time to occur. The role of the leadership will be that of guide, information giver and gentle co-ordinator of the meetings.

Designing a group calls for a good knowledge of what different group set-ups can achieve, and it is a lack of this kind of knowledge which tends to make people throw a group together on the assumption that it will work out all right when everybody meets. This haphazard approach may be successful, sometimes astonishingly so, but it is usually no credit to the leadership if it is.

It is simple to say that people's needs are different and therefore the ways in which those needs are met should match those differences. In essence this is what should be aimed for, but in practice it is seldom easy to achieve.

Example

A group was established in a prison for inmates who were isolates. The planning for the group suggested a careful screening of the possible members: a closed group numbering no more than seven or eight in size. The original design proposed that the group should last six weeks, meeting on a weekly basis, and that the leadership would be directive, based on the fact that the group members would be likely to need a great deal of security. Other design factors included the level of ability of the members to express themselves, similarity of intelligence levels, and stable social backgrounds.

Many factors were considered in the design of this group, but one above all the others proved to have been wrongly assessed. This was the factor of time. In practice, dealing with the problem of isolation takes far longer than six weeks at one meeting per week; six months would be a more reliable estimate. The social elements which bring about the isolation of individuals within a community are neither simple nor tractable.

When a group has been thought about, then the acts of creating it entail a certain amount of responsibility. After all, if the thought to create a group had never occurred, the group would never have come into existence, and by any standards that must mean that some responsibility arises for seeing that the creation operates reasonably efficiently and without causing harm to anyone.

Some organizations recognize that the skill of group leadership is a very important one, and they tend to set up or use existing methods of training. Leaders created in this way are usually referred to as 'designated', which only means that they are provided by some social agency and that they have some understanding of the processes involved. The title also serves to distinguish them from leaders who arise from within some already existing group structure or who set about the business of creating a specific group on their own initiative. Such leaders are often described as 'natural' leaders.

Neither of these titles actually defines the way in which the leader will operate. This is usually more a matter of personal choice or is dictated by the exigencies of a situation. For instance, with a collection of people who know nothing about groups other than from their own life experience, a leader may decide that until the members of such a group become more aware of what is involved in being members of a group, s/he will have to assume a directive role. That is, s/he will have to guide, to set tasks and to develop the growing skills of the members.

It is not a particularly fruitful idea to think that individuals can be self-directing without some help in first recognizing what such a way of behaving actually entails. Children tend to like and need a sense of security, which comes from understanding where they stand in relation to other significant people in their lives. Such a basis gives them plenty of opportunity to experiment and test what is possible. The same is true of adults too, especially those who, for some reason or other, have not developed or had the chance to develop effective social skills and coping behaviours. This does not mean that such people should never be offered the opportunity to develop the ability to become self-sufficient. In fact, quite the reverse is true. But the development should be allowed to grow in conformity with the needs of those involved and not imposed as part of some philosophy which sees self-direction as a desirable end in itself without reference to the needs of members or of their ability to sustain such an approach.

WORKING WITH GROUPS

Group leadership can be directive; it can also be facilitative, enabling, a resource pool, or play any one of several other roles. The main factor must be that the role which any leadership takes on is appropriate to the situation of the group and of the abilities and experience of the members and of the outcome which the group holds as its essential aim. It must also be appropriate to the abilities of the leader.

Directive leadership

It is interesting to note that despite the social work credo, which lays great emphasis on individuals in the social work situation being able to be self-determining, there is a great predominance of groups which are leader-directive. I believe the reason for this is that directive leadership, which is essentially a controlling situation, feels safer and much less threatening than the more permissive forms. While this is indeed so, as we shall see in a moment, the situation is one which unless truly understood by those employing a directive form of leadership can slide imperceptibly into coercive and oppressive forms. Why is this so?

Well, one of the main problems that anyone wishing to work with groups has to face is that the leadership is always outnumbered by group members. This alone can pose a threat, so it is sometimes met by the leadership's assuming and hanging onto the control of the group in order to maintain a position of some advantage and to minimize the threat implied by sheer numbers. Such a posture often shows up quite clearly in groupwork beginners and has the effect of making the leadership that much less sensitive to the other people in the group. If leaders are devoting energy and attention to evolving a position of some security, there is less attention and energy left to devote to the group members. There is also the fact that such behaviour is quite easily spotted by group members, who see persons who are allegedly quite knowledgeable about groups behaving in protective and guarded ways, and accept this as a role model and set about protecting themselves.

In directive groups the position of leader is one of power. This assertion has been questioned many times by group leaders who have told me that they do not regard themselves as people of power. But the problem is not how the leader feels but how s/he is seen by the group members. That perception of power is an instrument of great use provided it is not abused – that is, inflicted on members who are already relatively powerless in order to keep them in that state. The exercise of this power must be justified in the sense that through the medium of its use information, knowledge, guidance and development can be created and the power of the members enhanced in dealing with the group and their problems themselves. Therefore what a leader does can be very significant. What a leader states to be his/her mode of behaving within the group and what the members actually see as behaviour need to be as consonant as is humanly possible. For instance, if the leader is unable to behave in the open and honest way which s/he has set as a mode of behaviour for the group, that leader will have grave difficulties in getting any of the members to behave in open and honest ways.

The role of central person

One of the roles which a leader can be seen to be occupying fairly frequently is described as that of 'central person'. If we think of the hub of a wheel, the focal point about which everything else revolves and, more importantly, to which everything is positionally related in a fixed order, then the centrality of the leader's role should be clear. It is an important concept for a whole variety of reasons, some of which we can discuss here.

If a group has been created by the operation of the leader, who first sees the need for a group and then sets one up, all the members will usually have been approached before the establishment of the group on a one-to-one basis by the leader in an attempt to put forward the value that a group could have for that person. Thus when the group convenes for its first meeting as a group, the one relationship which all the potential members have in common will be that which they have established with the leader during the setting-up procedures. Of course, other common relationships may also exist, depending on the nature of the selection of group members.

This common relationship is a key point. It cannot have escaped notice that groups tend to identify similarities and that in the early stages of the development of a group, similarities can be reassuring. People form clubs, select friends, and choose to work with others on the basis of perceived similarity if they are fortunate enough to be free to do so. Similarity and complementarity tend to make life easier and more rewarding. One of the great advantages that groups have is that they can offer the possibility of discovering that other people have the same or similar problems, have produced similar responses, and are usually pleased to meet others in the same boat for the comfort it offers of not being too different, isolated or compelled to struggle alone, often with inadequate resources.

Much else can stem from the central person role of a group leader, and it behoves any person convening a group in this way to recognize that it creates the possibility of this kind of perception of a relationship. Tied very closely to this may also be perceptions of power, either based on the assumption of the possession of expertise or emotionally based on the assumption of the ability to protect. As I suggested elsewhere, such perceptions *arise whether the leader intended that they should or not*, and to deny that they exist because they were not intended is to disparage the reality of the members and to belittle their perceptions as unworthy of consideration. It is necessary to accept that perceptions might have occurred and to say so, to check out to what extent they have actually occurred, and to decide how inimical, if at all, they are to the proposed developments of the group.

Of course, leadership responsibility is usually very high in the initial stages of a group, when some central power has to operate to set things up even if it has the form of being a committee. This can all change later as things become more settled. But many promising groups have been either retarded or destroyed by the initiating leader's being too ready to hand over responsibility for the group's welfare and direction long before it was either ready or wanting to take on such tasks. Thus the central person gambit is custom built to generate exactly the kind of attitude which will allow the leadership to exercise careful responsibility in the initial establishing period of the life of a group.

Like all exercise of power, it can be overdone and the scene may be set for domination by the leader, and maybe also for the establishment of an oppressive regime. If a leader believes that the exercise of personal power is essential for the welfare of the group, then this becomes a conscious leadership decision. But if this occurs through insensitivity to the situation, then a problem will have been created for the time when change to a less directive approach may be not only desirable but essential for the group's well-being.

Of course, if the original thesis was to set up a group with an intended directive leadership, e.g. in an area of treatment, with all the implications of the need for superior knowledge being applied for the benefit of others, then the central person form of establishing a group gets it off to the right kind of start.

One other possible form of this kind of approach merits attention here. The power which the central person may be perceived as possessing is by no means always the same, and does not need to be. Some paternalistic group leaders are seen as being essentially wise and understanding, some as charismatic, others as possessing authority which has obviously been vested in them by a higher body because of their skill or personality, all of which is bound up with credibility.

Now, there is a very strong need for any group leader to recognize how s/he is perceived by the group's members because, although that view may be different from the leader's, and even unacceptable, for them it is reality, and all the leader's actions and their responses will be interpreted in the light of it. Many times after working long hours with groups of people I have found them saying that it had taken them quite some time to get used to me as a person working with them and that I was not what they had supposed me to be by reputation. I am always chagrined on such occasions that I have not had the wit to recognize these feelings earlier and respond to them so that the group members could have been adjusted to the reality of the situation. I might add that one reason for these incidents is that they occur among groups of people usually so competent and well adjusted that either it is very easy to forget, or it seems ludicrous to suppose, that amongst such people these attitudes can exist.

The role of central person is unique and it offers an opportunity for a leader to move fluently in any one of a number of major directions. Like everything else connected with groupwork, the essential basis is recognition: seeing what has happened and being aware of it, no matter how dotty it may appear to be. One of the phrases I realize I have used most often to people learning about groups is that they must 'blow their minds' – in other words, widen the basis of their reception of behavioural patterns and be prepared to accept what at first blush appears unusual as very probably correct.

Enabling

The concept of the role model is very important in group leadership. Without question, telling people that they should behave in a particular way is one of the least effective methods of getting them to behave in that way. If individuals can see that they stand to gain either in prestige or by increasing their satisfaction in some way, then they will be prepared to make changes in their behaviour towards the required patterns. If they can be shown by demonstration or the pointing out of examples that the behaviour in question does actually bring about desirable results, there will tend to be a strong incentive to adopt the behaviour demonstrated.

Enabling is a process of guiding, of encouraging, of showing the consequences of behaviour patterns and of asking whether this is what was intended; of making visible behaviour which is beginning to show understanding of what is required and of deflecting the effects of bad behaviour to protect those liable to be hurt, but always making specifically clear what is going on. It cannot be stressed too often that if a group leader sees it as part of his/her brief that the members shall be enabled to take some understanding and power to influence the group into their own hands – that they shall come to know and recognize what is going on – then that leader has to initiate a pattern of behaviour which makes everything explicit by verbalizing what s/he sees and checking that with what the members see.

Many people in a group will see something happen and say nothing about it because they are not accustomed to commenting on social behaviour in unfamiliar surroundings. They may make an assumption that there will be no need to comment as everyone else in the group will have seen it too. But, of course, this is not true. And even if the other group members have seen it, they will most likely not have seen it in the same way. Group members have to learn this, just as they have to learn that there is a need to display how they feel and how they are responding to what is going on more in this situation than they might in 'real life' outside the group. In this way, members can grow in awareness of the way in which their feelings and thinking compare with those of others in the group. The sense of sharing and understanding begins to develop, and eventually a level of trust will stem from this which will allow the group to begin to work as a unit.

Co-leadership or partnership

Group leadership has the potential to be an occupation which tends to generate a considerable amount of anxiety when practised by an individual. Consider that, if for no other reason than that a single leader is always outnumbered by the group members, there is the possibility of such an individual feeling overwhelmed should the group display a consensual antipathy. But apart from this, there is also the problem for a single leader of having to try to handle the two main aspects of leadership at the same time. If s/he becomes engrossed in the business of the group, its task and in the processes of decision-making, then s/he may well not be able to see how the emotional aspects of the group are developing. Where there are two leaders acting in close co-operation and understanding of one another's behaviour patterns, these tasks can be shared. The feedback that each can give the other is valuable in that it can often reveal aspects of leadership and other behaviour which had previously gone fairly unrecognized.

But co-leadership or partnership needs to be explicitly prepared for, and an agreement between partners reached as to how they are going to work together. They also need to be well aware of how each tends to work in groups, and above all, what their principles and beliefs are about the group-work process. If this preparation is done well, then the partnership can act as an effective role model of various aspects of relationships that work for the group – for instance, as examples of gender relationships, of racial, age and personality factors; of a relationship in which can be seen equality of status, of sharing, and of visible differences working in harmony. Such a relationship can take advantage of the different skills that each partner has to offer; their different knowledge, aims and aspirations, and their ability to share. But I must stress that with the best will in the world such an effective partnership needs to be worked at assiduously well before it is exposed to the observation of a group. It is well not to forget that there is much recorded evidence that the perceptions of group members of their group leaders are often significantly different from those the leaders hold of themselves. Where group members are seeking for reassurance in the way that their leaders behave, unresolved differences between those leaders are, or can be, generators of suspicion and inhibit the development of trust.

Thus consultation and a frank exchange in planning beforehand and an equally open and careful assessment period after group sessions is an essential part of the development of an effective working leadership partnership.

Because there tends to be a lack of training for groupwork leadership, co-leadership presents the possibility of a kind of apprenticeship for learners. Such a process with a skilled leader can highlight difficult issues, show what sharing responsibility is actually like, and offer first-hand experiential learning of coping skills. It can also offer support in an otherwise very exposed situation and supply an increase in resources both for the group and for the apprentice groupwork leader.

General dispersed leadership

Essentially, dispersed leadership takes place in those groups where no one person has what might be called a steady leadership function. In these situations, leadership functions are taken by consensus, or allocated in general discussion on the basis of a willingness of the electee to perform, or by virtue of his/her appearing to possess the requisite skills or knowledge to do so. Such leadership is held only by agreement with the group and the individual concerned, and is relinquished when the specific need for it has passed.

It can be a method of using the resources of group members very fully, as for instance in a group of professionals who are very clear about the individual skills they possess and who are sufficiently trusting of each other not to be obstructive or jealous. Without the clear knowledge of skills, such a group can become somewhat chaotic and have a low performance level.

Self-help group leadership

Self-help groups are also referred to as mutual aid groups and support groups.

> Modern self-help groups in the Western World are problem-focused, are established by people who share a problem, their raison d'être (and activities) focus around the problem, and people cease to belong when they perceive their problem solved or they no longer can benefit from participation in the group.
>
> (Lavoie, Borkman and Gidron 1994: 334)

The leaders of many such groups are the members of the group themselves. The groups can be national in scope or local or focused to a specific problem area. But in any case they are the extreme end of the continuum where leadership resides within the group. The processes which such groups develop are largely concerned with the offering of models; of mutual support; of the 'feel-good factor' which comes from being a helper rather than a victim; of the development of empathy or what has been called 'identification resonance' where there is little need of explanation because all fellow members know at first hand what is being talked about. Objectives of destigmatization and of empowering each other by a combinatorial process are also common in these groups.

Professional groupworkers have often been wary of self-help groups. But professionals can and do supply some very effective leadership skills. For instance, if they become convinced of the values of a particular group they can use their contacts to disseminate information and explanations. They can sometimes help such groups in their start-up procedures and act as initiators, suggest ideas and offer information. When the group is up and running, they can act as consultants and supervisors. These latter roles are a good example of facilitative leadership where experience is deployed from an external position without direct involvement or interference.

When a self-help group is prepared to offer a professional leader membership of the group, this is generally established as a partnership or a form of coalition and is done on the basis of an agreement which confirms the members' autonomy and independence, and decrees different spheres of influence and control.

As we have seen, there are many forms of leadership. What is essential is that whatever form leadership takes, it must be relevant to two very important and basic factors. It must first and foremost be relevant to the needs of the group members, and this means that over the life of the group it needs to change as those needs change. It must essentially be compatible with the personality, abilities and beliefs of the leader. It may be that because of the infinity of human problems some leaders will choose to operate only in clearly defined spheres and others will take on wider aspects. It is good to be able to be flexible but it is probably more important to know one's limitations and boundaries.

Stage-by-stage example

Introduction

It seemed to me that one of the best ways in which I could demonstrate some of the points I am trying to make would be to offer an analysis of a group situation in the hope that it would show clearly the step-by-step processes involved. I have chosen to use the example of a group of social work students for a whole variety of reasons. It takes the idea of group activity away from the field of therapy, where it has all too often reposed, and places it in the field of learning, which is much more appropriate for the kind of groupwork discussed in this book. It shows very clearly many of the constraints which affect the groupworker in general practice – for example, a pre-selected group, clearly defined time limits, breaks in contract and the embedded nature of most groups in larger organizations. It emphasizes many of the good points about groupwork, such as clarity of purpose, the function of leadership and the way in which a group changes over time. The various stages of the group are described at the end of Chapters 5–9, each stage being relevant to that particular chapter.

Stage 1: Conceptualization

I have always maintained that there is no real substitute for group experience. If one is going to learn how to work with people in a group, then it becomes essential that experience in a group is one of the major factors of preparation. It stands to reason that if the principal skills of a groupworker are of a practical nature, then theoretical knowledge is a point of departure and not the main point of arrival.

This being so, I have always tried to give students who were learning about groups the opportunity to work in groups and to use those groups as instruments for learning about groups in general and their own group behaviour in particular. When a group of students is large, this poses some problems, but where it is of the order of nine to fifteen, the solution lies in regarding the total number as the population of the group and in making the most of what this throws up in terms of the effects of size.

Let us now look at the logical sequence which follows:

1   The actual course contains a small number of students.
2   Part of the course entails learning about groups and how to work with them.
3   The need is to find the most effective way of achieving maximum learning, given the constraints of time, other demands, the environment, the potential of the group members, resources, etc.

Within the teaching system a group experience lasting over three terms is feasible. The theoretical inputs come partly from other sections of the course, partly from previous education and partly from being offered in the group as its members see some necessity for particular bits of knowledge to cope with situations in which they find themselves. Within the learning situation the group experience is compatible with the ethical and philosophical ideals of social work practice and will, I hope, demonstrate the effects of offering this kind of learning to people and the need for absolute sincerity in pursuing groupwork activities.

The responsibility for establishing the group lay clearly with me as teacher, and the general aims were reasonably well thought out and ready for presentation to the students so that a primary contract could be made. Then there was the need to look at the possible constraints to see how, as far as they were known, they could affect the group outcomes, and to evaluate past attempts at running a group in these circumstances, mainly to see what lessons could be applied to this new endeavour.

Constraints: the environment

The environment was generally conducive to this kind of learning except for the fact that the course norm of assessment of progress produced particular difficulties with the confidentiality of the group and rendered the development of trust between me as leader and the students as group members rather uneasy.

TIME

There were three main time factors:

1 the duration of sessions and the necessity of fitting in with a timetable involving a number of other people;
2 the frequency of sessions;
3 the amount of time when students were actually available. For example, such time was bounded by the length of term, placements and holidays.

RESOURCES

Rooms and equipment of suitable nature were no problem; the leadership skills available were, I think, adequate!

MEMBERS

Problems arose in terms of the group's composition because the potential members were already selected on criteria not entirely compatible with those which I would normally have used for entry to a specific groupwork course. But they were all social workers, and any expressed interest in groupwork came as a bonus. The membership did eventually pose some problems in terms of commitment, which had been expected. The learning potential was high. Previous experience of the members showed some similarities; educational backgrounds were also similar; attitudes to groupwork were very varied but the potential was good.

SIZE

This intake had nine students, well within the reasonable limits of a learning group. This fact alone was valuable as they tended to work together as a group not only during groupwork sessions but also for most of their academic time.

OPEN/CLOSED NATURE OF THE GROUP

This group was closed, apart from odd absences due to illness and other problems. The fact that the students became interdependent generated quite an intense group atmosphere.

SELECTION

Selection had already taken place, based upon criteria of acceptability for social work training and education, which were not necessarily the essential criteria for acceptance as students of groupwork.

ACTIVITY

The activity was open discussion but included role play, games, exercises and video-taping.

INTERVENTION

Initially, intervention was directive, but it became facilitative later as members became more aware of how the group functioned. The main purpose was to inspire the ability to observe and understand the processes which occur in groups.

CONTRACT

The primary contract was formed around the idea of learning *about* groups. Eventually this was modified by the group as the students became more aware of what there was to learn, and was based upon their particular choices. The only major constraint here was that of the learning focus of the course as a whole.

I recognize that this conceptualization is learning-specific, but the idea is not to offer a model to be followed exactly, but rather to show how in a particular situation the pattern of conceptualization worked out.

Part II

BASIC GROUPWORK

6

TURNING IDEAS INTO ACTION
Getting started

Once the idea has been conceived that a group may be an appropriate way of dealing with a particular problem or situation, the next important thing to do is to turn the idea into an action – that is, to start the process of bringing a group into being. In some ways this is a task of some difficulty for a beginner. Many people have absorbed the basic information about the ways in which groups of people behave, but interestingly enough, large numbers of these same people, while they have been members of many groups, may never have entered the business of actually starting a group from scratch. The opportunity may never have arisen; there may have been no encouragement from others; or there has never been enough time or available resources. There are a plethora of similar reasons why this should be so.

But much more likely than all of these is the well-known difficulty of all professional training of turning what is learned as theory into actual practice based on that theory. This problem is almost always made worse by a lack of any opportunity to try out newly learned ideas under the skilful and sympathetic guidance of someone who has experience and skill. Where such guidance is available, the results are usually quite remarkable, for two reasons. First, much confidence can be gained from being with someone who has apparently succeeded and who has garnered a considerable store of practical experience. Second, there is the availability of discussion when the learner is faced with difficulties.

In Chapter 3 we looked at some of the main ways in which groups originate. All these origins showed that at some stage the process of thinking and exploring had to be turned into making contact with people, not only those who would be directly involved as members but also those who might have some ability to influence both the establishment of a group and its future life.

It is often the case that people in authority do not actually understand what effects groups can have on the quality of life of their members, largely because administration tends to have goals and priorities in the allocation of resources that differ from the goals and priorities of those who work directly with people. The effectiveness of many groupwork projects

67

depends to a great extent upon the energy and goodwill of those involved at all levels.

An issue which I have had constant experience of, particularly in groups started in large organizations, is that there is a marked unwillingness, both on the part of those starting new projects and by those who have already had that experience, to compare and share information and ideas. It is almost as if there was being enforced a kind of copyright of ideas and experience, which means that individuals frequently have to set out to solve problems that have already been solved by others. When considered unemotionally, this represents a great waste of time and effort.

So the point must be re-emphasized that the establishment of a group takes place in an environment which will inevitably affect the possible outcomes of the group, and maybe even its viability. The degree of co-operation which is required from others in an organization and other agencies and communities who are involved, even if only marginally, means not only that they need to know what is being proposed but also that their help, or at least non-interference, would be desirable. This often requires some active proselytization on the part of prospective group convenors.

SELECTION

Selection is a thorny problem for several reasons. In classic group therapy practice, members of a prospective group have always been selected on some very obvious criteria, which has had the effect of producing a collection of individuals with some strong elements of character, need and problem which would be conducive to achieving successful outcomes for the group and its members. In the early days of groupwork practice this model was taken over by non-therapeutic groupworkers, with, in most cases, equal effectiveness. But as groupwork has spread to many different areas of human experience, this form has been found wanting, particularly when groups were self-selecting and also when the number of people available or suitable to become members was so small that choice, i.e. selection, could not possibly be an option.

One paramount fact emerges from any thorough consideration of this problem in selection. This is the essentially simple and obvious point that a group in which the members have been specifically selected to join the group because they are deemed to possess characteristics and abilities and experience which will be of benefit in the work which the group has to do will be a very different group, both in procedure and outcome, from one in which no such selection procedure was possible. For instance, those who practise groupwork with groups which already have an existence, such as families, gangs, work groups, etc., know that selection is not an option. Instead they have to work with patterns of behaviour which exist within the group and which beyond doubt originated so that the group could perform its established function. Usually, by a process of highlighting those patterns for the group members a groupworker can bring into focus why the group may not be fulfilling its functions as well as it might, or show that the ends which are being attained are not particularly socially acceptable.

In essence, selection is a form of manipulating some of the constraints which operate on a group to reduce those with negative effects and promote those which are deemed to be positive.

In any event, selection is a risky procedure because the ability to assess the potential any member may have for any particular group is not an exact science. The process has even more dimensions of risk currently because individuals have a heightened awareness of their particular needs and of those processes of selection which might be regarded as discriminatory. Thus particular care must be taken when group members come from different ethnic communities unless the group is specifically designed to deal with such difference – with mixed race, sex, age of members – unless a specific agenda of exploring difference for such a group is its main reason for existence.

The problem is not one just found in multiracial groups in which black people are in a minority. In such circumstances, as Bandana Ahmad (1990: 62) writes, 'Black members, instead of gaining support and strength, instead of sharing common feelings and aspirations, have found themselves even more isolated and sometimes in threatening conditions', a process usually described as marginalization. Problems are also found in groups where the balance between black and white is equal. There may be differences in perception about some issues which confound a sharing of experience, a difference in priorities so great that unrewarding conflict is inevitable.

Most of us are faced with little or no room to select. There are either too many people or too few for what we have worked out as the optimum number for the particular group we want to run. In many cases the number of people available has been arrived at by criteria which have little relevance for groupwork purposes. For instance, groups of students on social work courses have been selected not on the basis that they will be able to work together but only because of the fact that they satisfy the entrance criteria of the particular institution to which they have applied and that there are vacancies for them. A group pre-selected on non-groupwork criteria then has to be considered as containing, or as being subject to, extra constraints, and the effects these will have on the group's performance need to be considered very carefully. Some aims might now be impossible of achievement, so that others might have to be substituted.

Many examples of the problems of selection can be found in the literature of working with groups.

Example

A number of students on a social work course spent part of their time in a group situation where the basic purpose was to use their observations of their own group to learn about the processes which are general to all groups. The students had been selected for the course in the first instance not on their ability to work in groups but on criteria associated with being able to become competent social workers. The kinds of difficulties they experienced in learning to work together as a group were in no small measure due to the fact that the selection process had not created any immediately obvious bonds between them. So, much of their time in the first few weeks of being in the group was devoted to discussing norms and standards and the structure of their group. This is a classic sign of the kind of anxiety when group members are unsure of what is expected of them and thus of their safety within the group. The development of trust, which is essentially based upon a first-hand familiarity with the behaviour patterns of others which allows a degree of reasonably accurate prediction, took place over that time and led to the diminution of security-oriented behaviour and cleared the way for the group to get down to some really productive work.

Some groups when working together to learn the skills of working with people have been selected on the basis of the job they already occupy. If they then decide to use a special and different form of group to enhance their learning situation, for example some form of sensitivity training, many factors may mitigate against such an exercise becoming a success. In the first instance, many individuals will be there who have no wish to be part of such an exercise, having some fear of what is involved. Even if ground rules are made with the express purpose of protecting these people, the group is not likely to have a great deal of success because not all the people present in the group were selected on the basis of being involved in sensitivity training.

This is a special case of a very much more common occurrence in group-work – that is, when groups are formed of individuals who have little desire to be present in such a group but are there because the alternative methods of their disposal are considered to be worse. Probation officers are frequently faced with this form of selection, when there are a given number of probationers available who have committed various but similar offences and groupwork has been recommended in an effort to change their behaviour patterns, or at least make them more conscious of the consequences of their patterns of behaviour.

Another form of limited selection occurs when groupworkers take over already established groups, such as gangs or families, where no selection is possible. Such situations highlight very clearly the need of the worker to be as sure as is humanly possible of what s/he is trying to do, because only then will it be possible to make a reliable estimate of how far the constraints imposed by the prior existence of the group will affect the desired outcome.

CLARITY OF PURPOSE

It is essential that the purpose for which a group is established should be clear – at least, as clear as it is possible to be, given the circumstances in which the convenor finds him/herself. This helps to make the establishment of any kind of group a very logical process.

If the necessary thinking, discussion, preparation and exploration have taken place, then the worker is in the position of being able to present to the potential group members a package which s/he has the advantage of knowing inside out. It is still, however, unquestionably true that when the convenor is faced with selling this package and answering questions about it, gaps in the preparation can readily become exposed. The idea that people should share problems, skills or knowledge is not one which is readily accepted in Western society, except in clearly defined areas of everyday life such as clubs and families and friendship groups; the idea will have to be sold. It is possible to obtain co-operation for one-off events much more easily than for the extended period of time required for a group. Of course, where people are, as it were, drafted into a group as a condition of, say, a probation order, then the selling process has to take place much more directly, not just in terms of what may be gained, but also in terms of consequences and alternatives.

But in any case, whether a group leader takes over an existing group or attempts to create one by selecting individuals to comprise it, s/he is faced with the need to explain clearly what s/he is about and to obtain the consent, however grudging, of those involved at least to give it a try. We have seen earlier how in the concept of 'central person' a particular relationship of members to the leadership can begin to develop as a result of this exercise.

CONTRACT

Frequently the discussion which takes place about joining a group or about the use of an existing group for a new purpose (for example, using the family group as a vehicle to examine its own processes) is referred to as forming the basis of a primary or initial contract, or at least as a working agreement. But it is essential to say at this stage that such agreements need to be given very careful consideration, and it must never be forgotten that although the group-workers involved will have a very clear idea of what is being asked, the members, although they may understand the words of what is being suggested, may have little appreciation of what translating those words into behaviour will actually imply. But nevertheless the whole idea of contract is based upon the approach to co-operation between individuals, which means that it is best obtained by securing a commitment to be involved based on as good an understanding of what is involved as it is possible for them to achieve.

In many cases the first contractual obligations may be just that the individual approached will think about what is being offered and will be free to offer suggestions and comments and able to seek reassurance about any points not understood or which are bothersome. Of course, some people are requested to join groups as part of a contractual obligation already in place. For example, a psychiatrist may use groups as part of his/her treatment plan, and patients may be expected to attend as part of their treatment programme. Refusal in these circumstances may be deemed to constitute a breach of a medical contract, with the possibility of that patient being dropped from that programme.

A contract is a working agreement between the group leadership and the potential or actual members of a group. It has several very important functions, not least of which is to register the varied expectations of the parties to the group and their commitment to it.

When a collection of people gather together in a group there may well be an assumption on everyone's part that as they are all reasonably intelligent they will all have roughly the same idea of why they are there. Usually nothing could be further from the truth. Each and every person, however much publicity has been put out beforehand, however much information has been given on a personal basis, will have assimilated only that part of it which appears to relate to that individual and to his/her previous understanding and ideas and beliefs. This being so, there is a disparity of expectations which can be quite great and which, if not taken into account, will create the possibility of high levels of disappointment and frustration for many of the members.

How can a contract help with this problem? Quite simply, by asking everyone involved to spell out what they think they are meeting in the group to do. This applies to children as well as adults, to those who are not expected to have any ideas as well as to those who have too many. This is not a foolproof method, for there are those who have ideas but, for a whole variety of reasons, have little or no ability to express them.

Clearly, from a group leader's point of view a contract places a great burden on him/her to know exactly what s/he has to offer, even though it may be incomplete and tentative. This means that such a leader will need to have thought through the available reasons for starting this group. It is more than likely that this will lead to the leader knowing that s/he is not entirely sure of what s/he wants to achieve, and this should be enshrined in the leadership side of the contract. S/he will suggest that by working together they will be able to use their different skills and abilities not only to further the aims of the group but also to amend them in the light of increasing understanding – unless the group is essentially to be directed by the leadership, in which case the leadership's suggestions, based on expertise and experience, will have much more force. But whatever the leadership form it is incumbent upon the leaders, if they have clear ideas of what may be required, that these should be stated, including as precise a statement as is possible of what they, the leadership, can bring to the situation.

Most prospective group members will have their own ideas about what they want out of the situation, even if these are not coherently structured. They must be encouraged to say what these ideas are because it will soon be obvious that not everyone has similar ideas, and a certain amount of bargaining will need to take place if enough areas of sufficient satisfaction for the members are going to be covered.

As I have already hinted, a very important part of the operation of a group contract is that it should be flexible. No one can be prescient enough, even with a wealth of experience, to be sure how things are going to work out, though the more experience there is available, the better the idea of what might occur can be. Thus a contract which is rigidly maintained from the starting point of the group is liable to be one which less and less fits the needs of the group, unless the group actually stagnates.

At the beginning, therefore, it is advisable to indicate that the contract being made is modifiable as the group grows and changes; that any such modifications are to be discussed and to be adopted only if there is a general consensus. If the group exists in an environment in which very firm rules about behaviour obtain, then the original contract should have included this fact as one of the immovable constraints within which the group will need to work. In some cases no amount of consensus about the need to change will be able to change the major constraints, but at least some discussion of them will ensure that their influence is clearly, rather than vaguely, understood.

Apart from being a working tool of great value in ensuring a high level of satisfaction and member participation, a contract clearly has a non-verbal contribution to make. It implies that one of the main learning purposes of the group is for the members, individually and collectively, to carry responsibility for their own actions and not to be dependent upon others. The whole of one of the most basic purposes of using groups – to help people to use the resources they possess, and can develop in conjunction with others – is underlined by the contract. It should be a clear statement of shared and co-operative endeavour.

All areas of the group's construction, running, purposes, etc., can be subjected to contractual agreement. Thus the very mechanics of the group – what time it will start, how long sessions will last, the duration of the group, its nature, the kind of activities and points of possible contention such as smoking, violence, the form of rewards and punishment for various kinds of behaviour – are all subject to contractual agreement within the reality of the constraints which exist, and within the competence and experience of the group leadership.

Example

A club had been formed by local authority social workers designed to be a place where people who had been in-patients of the local psychiatric hospital could meet once a week for social and recreational purposes. The contractual agreement made between the organizers and prospective members before they left hospital included also the suggestion that social work help would be available, but on request only. The club was therefore to be run by a committee of appointed members, and the social workers would operate as advisers and consultants if required. After a period of time during which the club ran very successfully, the contract was modified to include the provision of subgroups within the club structure, which would have a much more therapeutic and advisory nature as the members felt the need of them. The basic contractual obligations were discussed with the club as a whole as at that time constituted, and the conditions under which these subgroups would operate were drawn up. They became a successful feature of the club, but support for them tended to fluctuate as the membership changed over the years.

ACTIVITY CHOICE

One of the major areas of any contractual agreement will be to specify what activity a group will use to achieve its goals. Often enough, the very nature of the group will clearly indicate what this will be, though not so often clearly seen is the fact that the main function of the group and the kind of activities which serve to establish and maintain it in existence are not necessarily even similar.

Thus the establishment of most groups takes organizational skill, which involves propaganda, advertising, committee procedures, endless discussion, mediation, contact, etc. The group when established, depending on its nature, may require skills of a different order connected with a knowledge of the dynamics of groups and the ways in which these can be harnessed to fulfil the group's aims. It is not always possible to discover the two rather different sets of skills in one person. It may not even be desirable.

When people are asked what they think groups 'do', answers tend to vary from one extreme, that of talking, discussing, decision-making, to what are usually lumped together as 'activities' – that is, games, leisure pursuits and activities which have more of the feel of pleasure than of work about them. Of course this is true, but it is unfortunate that this concept of activities is so common. Thus most people are familiar with groups which are used for recreation and leisure purposes and perhaps less familiar with groups used for so-called 'serious' purposes, such as committees, decision-making bodies and forms of 'treatment'.

But familiarity exists with the idea that children can play in a group. Indeed, there has been a proliferation of such units, called playgroups. It is accepted that young people carry out quite a large number of their social activities in groups – but it is still a barely accepted idea that 'normal' adults might benefit from 'playing' in a group. My main points in making these comments are two:

1 The activity which is the main programme of the group can be selected from a wide spectrum of possibles. Its principal value must be only that it can actually help to achieve what the group is aiming at.
2 There is no valid reason why the activities performed by the group should necessarily remain the same throughout the life of the group.

Unusual situations cannot be well met just by discussing what is likely to happen. Much of the life of young people is concerned with attempting to cope with situations for which they are not usually well prepared – for example, job interviews, or relationships with adults in a work environment. Many inventive people give their ideas a dummy run, if they can, in which those ideas are tried and tested for practicality in conditions which are as near as can be to the real thing. Groups frequently find this not only hilarious but also a very useful thing to do. Situations can be practised in relatively 'safe' surroundings, and though they may have an air of artificiality about them, they can be very productive of much social learning.

Inevitably the understanding about the ways in which other people might feel and behave in a given situation can be increased. Also, there is the possible spin-off that learning about oneself will develop, because however 'artificial' the created situation may be, it is an interaction with 'real' people involved and thus contains many of the same ingredients as are found in normal social behaviour.

With children and young people, the difficulty of encouraging them to talk about their lives lies in the degree of their ability to conceptualize and abstract. This is even more difficult if long experience has made them not only bitter but suspicious with feelings that they always come out on the wrong end of any deal, however kind the intentions of those proposing it may be. This problem can sometimes be dealt with by removing the need to talk about the past and instead talking about something which is immediate and present, such as a game, an exercise, or some kind of physically involving performance with other group members which can then become the focus of discussion. Recency lends point to the discussion and it is not obviously connected to the problem areas, though these will affect relationships and will probably emerge in the talking about the activity.

This technique may sound somewhat devious, but it is essentially based upon two very important assumptions:

1   that the group members will gain some benefit from being able to talk about their problems and difficulties even indirectly, and
2   that if a direct approach is inevitably going to encounter resistance and generate resentment for many possible reasons, then bearing in mind the many ethical considerations involved and accepting that some form of help is necessary, it must be worthwhile to prepare people to receive the help they would otherwise reject for reasons that are not valid, being based upon ignorance, misunderstanding or conditioning.

Thus like most factors connected with work with groups, the activities that a group uses must be appropriate. Basically they should be adopted to achieve ends, empirically justified and within the abilities of the group members to use. Great care needs to be taken in the choice of activities because different ones produce different effects. Some activities separate individual from individual and need very careful handling to bring about the necessary integration and sharing so that what started out as separating becomes binding and group oriented. Nothing is calculated to use less of the dynamics of a group than activities which isolate and encapsulate the individual members so that, although they may be occupying contiguous space, they are hardly aware of each other's presence, and interaction between them is minimal.

I think that enough has been said to demonstrate that activity choice is very wide and certainly includes the possibility of co-operative work and of group living. The concept that a group is only a 'real' group when it is seriously discussing some fundamental issues of concern to its members must be dispelled to make way for one which indicates that there are many ways of using the dynamics of group interaction for the benefit of group members. I have many times suggested to groupworkers that they do not use effectively what creative imagination they possess but are too restricted in following precedent. The needs of group members change from generation to generation and their understanding of how to achieve their goals is based upon having experienced different social conditions. New ideas are needed to meet old problems which present in new and different forms backed by different belief systems. Caution is necessary, for an overflush of imaginative enthusiasm can produce a situation in which the activity becomes an end in its own right rather than the means to an end. There are occasions when this may be justified – in the use of a group to study its own procedures, for instance – but usually such an interest in an activity tends to produce a group which has lost its way and which then becomes stagnant as far as the productive use of the group processes is concerned.

It is very difficult to write about operating a group from the point of view of the leadership without unintentionally creating the impression that leaders need to be omniscient. Of course this is incorrect, but I would also like to stress that current society has turned so much away from the concept of excellence in trying to improve the lot of some sections of the community that it is in fair danger of discrediting any kind of skill whatsoever as being discriminatory or condescending in some way. But skill has to have its proper place in this context – that is, to be used to help to bring about circumstances which enhance the lives of all those concerned. In this context it is useful in the area of creating and of adapting existing groups to look at the leadership's responsibility in establishing the 'rules of the game' and then to look at what have been called 'ground rules'.

RULES OF THE GAME

It may sound a little facetious to be talking about a 'game' and its rules when concerned with something as serious as working with groups. But it is one way of indicating the difference, which is sometimes ignored, that can exist between the group leadership and the other members of the group.

If a group leader is experienced and knowledgeable in the matter of working with groups of people, then whenever s/he sets up a group s/he is in a position of some advantage as far as anything connected with a group is concerned over the other members – unless, that is, the group contains members who are also somewhat experienced in being in groups. It is commonly assumed that because we all live, work and play in groups, we all understand the workings of groups equally well. But this is obviously not true, largely because the fact that groups are everywhere accepted as a part of everyday life means that most of us do little thinking about how they operate but just accept them as part of the social furniture. This is where the analogy with games comes in as a simple illustration.

It is almost impossible to play even the simplest of games with any degree of success if the rules which govern it are unknown. This is almost exactly the state in which most people enter a created group. In any game situation those who know the rules try to instruct learners so that they can start to play the game with some confidence; so that what they are doing is not vitiated by being against those rules. As learners play longer they should in the natural course of events become more adept and able to employ their skill at the game within the rules; to be able to play creatively rather than obediently, to begin to be able to play for enjoyment and effect rather than just to learn.

The analogy with groupwork is close. If new members of a group are to be able to derive maximum benefit from that membership, in the end they will have to learn not only the rules but how to operate within them for their own and the group's ends. This means that the group's leadership, in order to teach the members how to tap the resources the group contains, will need to show them the rules of this particular game and stand by to see that the rules are learned and observed.

What are the rules of groupwork? Well, they are the ways in which experience and research have shown that members of a group can best co-operate in order to exercise influence; become aware of their own behaviour; acquire knowledge and understanding of how power is given and used; and learn how to use the resources of the group and others for individual and group benefit and how to benefit from the support and encouragement of membership. In other words, what the leadership should be trying to do is to show the membership how to get the most out of the group of which they are a part through a degree of procedural conformity.

GROUND RULES

The idea of 'ground rules' is somewhat similar to that of a basic contract except that it is usually the leadership, having wider experience and greater understanding of what has happened in past groups, who try to limit certain possibilities. It may be, for instance, that one of the ground rules should be that if anyone is being very hard pressed by other group members, that member can appeal to the leadership for help, or even that the leadership has the undisputed right to intervene to protect that individual.

In essence, ground rules are limitations or boundaries placed upon the group by mutual agreement at its beginning. There is, of course, a problem, as there always is when those with experience try to limit damage by suggesting rules of procedure, which is that they may well be asking members to agree to some things which they do not fully understand. Explanations and examples may moderate this situation but, as we have seen in matters of behaviour, they also can be misunderstood. It is a situation which can bring repercussions later when understanding has been enhanced by experience. But generally what is involved here is a code of acceptable behaviour which is set up in advance. Its main function is to give guidance and to relieve the anxieties of some members of a group who may be unsure of their commitment and worried about their personal safety.

Two real values of ground rules are:

1   They can serve to speed up the process of getting on with the group's task by providing an initial protocol.
2   They can provide a method of learning about a group before becoming involved in it – a kind of foretaste or preview.

Against ground rules is the fact, already stated, of their being accepted without true understanding of their implications, and allied to this is the fact that the agreement is a rational one and cannot really involve members at a feeling level. It is essentially an overtly preventive device.

Ground rules should of course be explicitly formed for the kind of work and the kind of membership the group is expected to contain. But some general areas which should always be covered concern:

- reasons for being present;
- the need for interaction, to listen and to give everyone space to express themselves;
- that violence, either physical or verbal, is forbidden except under very unusual circumstances;
- group leaders can protect and see that the less able members get their fair share of space and time;
- that honesty and sincerity are group virtues and pretending is not;
- that the limits of confidentiality need to be clearly defined and understood, and are absolutely reality based;
- that group decisions are a matter for all members of the group, not just the dominant few; and
- that differences of all kinds between members are an essential part of the group's resources and not a matter for the exercise of discrimination.

No doubt as groupworkers become more familiar with certain kinds of groups they will realize that some of these rules are more applicable than others and that they will need to produce new ones of their own which fit their situations more effectively.

Little has been said so far about psychological and sociological theories of the ways individuals behave in groups, or about the ways such conceptions may be used to attempt to understand such behaviour. There are several reasons for this. Theoretical understanding of human behaviour, by which I mean the constructed and consistent theories which have been propounded to be used as yardsticks to measure and understand actual behaviour, have the great failing that none of their precepts is actually susceptible of proof except those which are based in physiology and genetics. Statistical generalizations make useful guidelines, but the translation into the practical help that a groupworker will need has to be made on the basis of personal preference. What works for one does not necessarily work for another.

What is essential for beginners is the availability of practical data which possess that rare property of being sufficiently specific to actual situations to be useful and general enough to have common application. Usually this means what is often called 'practice theory', which is a collection of principles, precepts and empirical data about group behaviour formed from the reports over many years of those who work with groups. Its main value is that what tends to be recorded is that which occurs most frequently, and by implication there-fore it is about what is most likely to be encountered by learners. But it has no direction. For example, the fact that a group leader can know that to increase the number of members in a group, with other factors remaining unchanged, will most likely increase the number of ideas available and decrease the amount of time available to each member in which to express them, does not give the leader any directive as to when such a manoeuvre might be under-taken. Other factors have always to be taken into consideration, like what the group is trying to achieve and, more importantly, what unintentional effects the strategy might possibly activate.

Of course, right from the beginning any potential group leader must have some personal idea of how a group can be used to attain some ends, or s/he would not contemplate using one. Thus such a leader is very liable to have seen, heard, been in or otherwise known about some form of group, or to have received some information about groups from some source. All of us also have some criteria for the interpretation and understanding of the behav-iour of others that we encounter every day – the so-called intuitive psychology. These criteria may be explicit or almost totally hidden, according to our interests and experience. But most important is the amount of hard thinking we may have directed to the problem.

Given that a group is then created, the kind of leadership ideas which will be involved can range from a basic precept such as 'people are fundamentally friendly and if left alone will soon learn to work together' to a very detailed and precise theoretical formulation of human behaviour such as psychodynamic theory or the precepts of cognitive psychology. I do not mean 'precise' here in the sense of accurate, but in terms of the minutiae of the theory. In another sense, then, the possession of some concepts about human behaviour dictates the techniques which are used in the running of a group. The two major issues in this field have already been discussed in terms of whether the leader believes that s/he possesses most of the skills, knowledge and understanding and the group members little or none, or whether s/he believes that the major resources lie in the group and his/her business is to create opportunities for their recognition, development and use.

Let us take a very simple example of this. If the purpose of a group is to exchange information, then the relevant knowledge and skill in the group's leader should be around the knowledge of the ways in which people can absorb different kinds of information and how such absorption can be facil-itated. Thus if, as is commonly believed, people absorb information by having it presented to them clearly and efficiently, there is no problem. But the common belief is demonstrably untrue, especially where the information is either complex, unrelated to previous knowledge, or involves strong emo-tions. Other factors often involved are the relationships between the information givers and the receivers (for example, teachers have long known that if they are liked by their pupils, the latter will tend to work harder for them than they will for teachers they do not like); the effect of the environment; the degree of concentration possible; and the states of mind of the recipients and of their health.

Created and formed groups can exert a strong influence for conformity upon their members. This fact can be used in many different ways to enhance the take-up of learning. For instance, rewards for performance to the whole group can be withheld until all members have achieved essential standards. The pressure the group may then choose to exert upon the slower and less accomplished members can be quite great and may need monitoring. It is to be hoped that the pressure will be supportive and encouraging rather than punitive, and thus the individuals concerned can see how their accomplishments affect not just their own success but that of the whole group.

Stage-by-stage example

Stage 2: Creation

This section of the ongoing example, continued here from the end of Chapter 5, is devoted to describing how the learning group conceptualized at the end of the last chapter was brought into being.

The major problem was of course that the group as a collection of individuals already existed. So the creation of this group was really a matter of accepting that the selecting was done and of using all those processes which have been discovered to weld a collection of disparate individuals into a group unit. Time is of the essence in this operation as there is no way in which people can be forced into realizing that they need to trust one another even to the extent that would be appropriate for them to work together. Such a realization has to grow organically with the gradual accumulation of information gathered at first hand as to how people interact and where the acceptable boundaries are.

The first task was to explain what we were about from my point of view, I being the person with the most comprehensive overall view and experience. Then the students could say what they felt about the situation and what they understood was to happen, recognizing some very important factors. These were that their understanding of the situation and of the constraints of the environment and its relative unfamiliarty, being limited, would impose upon their freedom to express themselves initially. The element of uncertainty is always present in the first few sessions of any group, especially if it contains individuals whose experience of group life is limited or at least undigested. I don't doubt from my own experience of many years working in and with groups that this also applies to people with lots of time spent in groups.

81

From these very first explorations the possibility of a primary contract emerged – that is, I put as clearly as I could what I could offer the group, and what I expected from it. The students were encouraged to say what they felt they could offer and what they wanted from the group. As no really fundamentally irreconcilable desires emerged, we were able to form a basic contract around those areas on which we had mutual agreement, with a clear understanding that as the group progressed this initial contract could at any time be renegotiated. In this particular group of students there was a strong need to proceed slowly from the kind of learning they were used to as postgraduates to the more experiential form appropriate for learning about how groups work.

So our basic contract was founded on information first, with an obligation to review after a period of about four weeks, or earlier as required, to plan the next moves. This was well in accord with the principles of contract-making in that the element of change, as understanding increased, was built in. The students had to find out for themselves that the information they would receive could only be partly related to their previous learning and experience and that therefore some large part of it would not be of immediate or direct value. However, as the contract was formed, it enabled us to proceed and to start work together, especially as the contract also contained basic rules for behaviour and protection.

The relationship of the group members at this stage was clearly that of individuals to me as central figure, and the level of suspicion and caution was fairly high. This was shown in that my comments were sometimes interpreted as being devious and manipulative, and explanations of behaviour were constantly being demanded. Later in the group's life it was very interesting to hear the members relate what their feelings had been about this particular phase. But it is this kind of recall which allows both the members and the leadership to gain a good insight into the problems of starting a group, which otherwise might never have been particularly clear at the time of their occurrence or later and thus their impact probably underestimated.

This is also the time when testing-out occurred and most group members were trying to establish some understanding of the others without having to sacrifice too much of their own security in the process. The relationships which already existed between some members of the group before coming to the course were much used during this period and had to stand a great deal of strain. Because most of the students were family members with other responsibilities, they had a strong motivation not to remain in each other's company longer than was absolutely necessary. This also could have been responsible for the delay in developing higher levels of trust, and, as we shall see later, had to be dealt with by the group themselves when they recognized what this pressure was doing to their attempts to integrate as a unit.

By the end of the period stipulated as input by the primary contract, the group requested three things very close together: first, that a more experiential form of learning should replace the input sessions; second, that more time should be devoted to the sessions; and third, that they should be held in a room which was more conducive of closeness than a lecture room. The basic contract was modified accordingly, the requests acceded to and the first obvious signs of the group growing together had appeared as had the realization of how group pressures could develop.

7

THE MORE IMPORTANT STEPS
IN WORKING GROUPS

Once a group has been set up, the next issue is how it is going to run. This is really a matter of the directions in which those who have invested time and energy in setting up the group wish to take it, and their understanding of what they and the group as a whole want to achieve. Just as important is their understanding of how groups can function and what sort of influence and in which direction they will need to try to exert it, even if they are apparently committed to letting the group find its own way.

This chapter has been called 'The more important steps in working groups' for the simple reason that I think it is possible to define those areas of working with groups which if not appropriately handled can diminish quite markedly the chances of the group's being a success. Perhaps the most important are, first, the ability to see what is going on; second, the ability to decide what needs to be done, if anything, and how to do it; and third, the ability to assess the effect of what has been done.

THE ABILITY TO SEE WHAT IS GOING ON

Society tends not to put much of a premium on the ability to see what is going on under our very noses. The trouble with things like identity parades (mistaken identifications which have cost people their liberty) and the use that television and film can make of ambiguities are examples. The culprits are lack of attention, absorption in something else, habit and routine behaviour. We tend to see sufficient of our surroundings and the behaviour of others to enable us to pursue our daily business and it is only when a crisis strikes or when we have time to relax and stare that it becomes possible to realize just how much is actually going on to which we habitually pay little attention.

Now, the ability to observe is actually very important when working in and with groups. In an interview situation it is usually necessary to keep tabs on only one person, and this becomes fairly easy because attention is not divided and there is no need to have to make decisions about which person to look at. In a group, exactly the reverse is the case. There are several people who are

84

part of the group unit, not just one; they are all more or less involved and they are all able to influence what the group is doing. For a leader, then, and for members as well, it becomes essential that some kind of oversight should be kept.

The difficulty of doing this becomes immediately obvious when one tries to put such an oversight into practice in an actual group. I have repeatedly said to potential groupworkers that they should not concentrate on the person who may be talking, at least not all the time. If you want to see what effect the speaker is having on all the others present, then you must pay some attention to them. It is difficult. We seem to be conditioned to control conversations by looking at and looking away from someone with whom we are speaking and to concentrate on not missing the non-verbal cues which when read add very much more meaning to the actual verbal content.

If this is true of the immediate behaviour of individuals, and it is, then it is much more difficult to look at and *see* the larger effects their behaviour is having on the rest of the group. It is axiomatic that what is not seen cannot be taken into account, and very often, by not noting the effects individual members are having on their group, developments in group behaviour appear to have arisen out of the blue.

Example

In a group of ex-psychiatric patients who met regularly once a week for support in the business of readjusting to life outside a hospital environment, there were two who had said very little despite all the encouragement that the group leader, a social worker, could give. Then one week both these people had something to say, and the groupworker encouraged them to say it. The dialogue went on for a long time and eventually the group finished its session with hardly anyone else having said anything at all.

The following week, before the group started, the groupworker was reminded by at least two of the other members that they were also part of the group, and, pleased though they had been to see the two quiet ones begin to contribute, they did not want to sit all evening just listening to them again.

The larger effect of the two quiet ones had escaped the attention of the worker in his enthusiasm to encourage their participation. If he had been monitoring the interaction of the group as a whole, it would surely not have escaped his notice that the attention of the others had decreased, which in return reduced the level of their satisfaction in being in the group. It could be argued that the members had a responsibility to have broken up the dialogue themselves, but perhaps they had not reached the level of confidence or trust in the group which would have enabled them to take the risk.

It is not an exaggeration to say that effective observation is the basis of all successful work with groups. It is common experience to look at things and people without really seeing them. When we do see, it is often more likely that what we see will be what we expect to see rather than what objectively exists. We are likely to see what we have learned we are likely to see under given conditions. For instance, we are quite likely not to recognize familiar people if we come in contact with them in unusual situations where we have no expectation of seeing them.

This means that if a groupworker is going to be able to see what takes place in a group session, then s/he is going to have to remain consciously aware of not operating under normal conditions and to make a real effort of will to maintain an expanded level of observation. This implies contravening the convention of not being seen to be watching people: concentrating attention outside the self, watching what is being *done*, and trying to estimate the nature of the effects which are being produced in the group. These are all ways in which this new learning can begin to develop.

In the last sentence the word 'done' was emphasized, and it is now necessary to explain why.

Content and process

In the necessary observation of what goes on in a group, there are many areas of our past experience and learning and conditioning which we have to put to one side, largely because some of this past learning will probably obstruct our vision of what it is essential to see clearly. So we need to come to the difference between 'content' and 'process' and to show why it is necessary to emphasize the latter rather than the former, which is already a well-developed interactive habit.

Everyone knows what a process is, but it is still very difficult to describe simply. A process is something which is going on. It involves the changing of something into something else. It is dynamic and it usually produces an outcome which is different from what existed at the point at which it was first applied. For instance, the application of heat to uncooked food is a process, the process of cooking. It changes basic materials from one form into another.

In a successful group, process (or, more realistically, several processes – see Chapter 4) operates to change basic raw materials – that is, the individual members – by generating a situation in which the members gradually become a functioning unit and thus gain access to resources which were not available to them before. This is simple enough, but as I hinted above, all large processes seem to be almost endlessly composed of smaller processes which contribute to the larger effect. Thus the overall *process* of the group is brought about by a series of smaller processes which take place, such as the interaction between members and the development of acceptable ways of behaving in a particular group situation.

On the other hand, by 'content' is meant not what the group is 'doing' but what the members are saying, and this poses a problem. Western society is 'verbally oriented'. That is, we invest a great deal in the words we use and have a kind of implicit belief that by talking, everything in the world can be explained and understood. Words have a fascination, and there are still hints in our usage that words can possess the power in their own right to change things. There seems to be a widespread but erroneous belief that by using them in the 'right' way we can make other people understand the most abstruse ideas and feelings. To counter this, it is only necessary to note the exasperation many people experience when they realize that despite having spoken clearly and with thought, they are not understood. The problems inherent in ordinary communication are dealt with elsewhere in this book. Here I am concerned only with the fascination with verbal expression and the consequent difficulty of paying attention to anything else.

When a group is talking – that is, when members are speaking and being responded to – those involved tend for the most part to listen to the words which are being used and, if they are specifically looking anywhere, it will tend to be at the person who is speaking. This is not to deny that a large number of non-verbal clues such as expression, gesture, tone of voice, etc., are also being picked up and used in interpretation of what is being said. They are reinforcers of the message, and sadly are often missed when a serious conversation takes place without them, as for instance over a telephone line. However, at the same time many other things are going on. For instance, members of the group are observing rules of behaviour; they are thinking and establishing preferences; they are consolidating roles and performances by behaving as good people, as powerful or weak people, as angry or complacent people, and so on. In other words, all the factors referred to earlier as group processes are taking place and they all have as a common currency exchange the words and interactions which are being deployed.

A major problem for anyone wishing to work with and in groups has now been exposed. It is language. Words fascinate, and they draw a great deal of attention. But if we pay too much attention to the intended meaning of the words, then the processes of which they are part – the behaviour and interrelation patterns – will tend to occur unnoticed. It is axiomatic that in order to influence the business which a group is doing it is essential to *know* what that business actually is and how it is being performed at any given moment – what is being caused to happen by what is being said. If these indicators are missed, then it is almost certain that patterns of group behaviour will develop for which no explanation is readily available.

Such is our fascination with verbal exchanges, especially on subjects of immense personal interest. When one person speaks in a group, most of those present will tend to look at the speaker, seeking those non-verbal clues to sincerity, feeling, etc., which will aid in the understanding and interpretation of what is being said. However, a group leader or member who is interested in discovering what effect the speaker is having on fellow group members needs to pay less attention to the speaker and much more to everyone else. After all, words can be heard, whereas the behaviour of others has to be seen. The reactions of the others will often demonstrate very precisely what is happening in the group, and that exposure of the workings, the dynamics, of the group is the primary goal of anyone who aspires to enable a group to function effectively.

As accurate and as effective observation as is possible depends also on the kind of checking a leader or member is prepared to do. If assumptions about what is happening in a group are not checked out, then idiosyncratic bias will inevitably accompany individual interpretation, with the possibility that actions based upon those assumptions will be at best only partially effective.

Thus the leader who thinks that his/her group is not working and that it is in fact resisting the idea of working can take action on that belief. However, such a leader would be well advised to check with the group by a simple process of offering to the group his/her assumptions that such a state exists, and to check how close a fit they are with the group's perception of what is happening. It can be quite shattering on occasions like this to find that one's perception of the state of the group bears little resemblance to what the other members are seeing and feeling. There are many times, however, when the feelings and perceptions of the leader and others are an accurate reflection of what the rest of the group is seeing and feeling too. It can be gratifying to realize that the latter situation tends to become more prevalent after a great deal of time spent with groups, when experience begins to count.

Co-leadership, as we have seen earlier, is an extremely effective way of leading groups, and in particular in this instance of getting feedback on one's performance as a leader, especially in the way one either did or did not note changes in the group's behaviour through being over-involved in a particular part of it.

When groups are used as a means of exchanging ideas and for their members to talk freely with one another, the circle is the most appropriate formation for the group to use. There are, of course, very simple practical reasons for this, as we shall see shortly, but the circle, as a shape, has come to have a significance beyond these practical issues. For instance, it is said to represent democracy in that a circle has no definite head or tail and so the leader is seen to be equal to the other members and they to him/her. But it is only too certain that a very dominant personality can make his/her presence felt and control the proceedings just as well in a circle as in any other group formation.

There is an element of truth in the idea of the inherent democracy of a circle, but the main reason for discussion groups to sit in a circle is much more practical. If the members of a small group are going to interact freely with one another, they need to be able to see one another without any undue amount of changing positions every time they want to say something or to be able to see the expressions on their fellows' faces while they are saying it. It is not an accident that such groups have usually been designated face-to-face groups. Quite simply, the range of vision of the human eye is restricted. What is directly in front of us can be seen quite clearly, whereas objects to the side are less clearly defined. This sixty-degree cone of vision which is available when the head is held rigid allows only large objects and movement to be seen at the periphery of our field of vision, and even those with some loss of clarity. Sitting in a circle makes the most of this cone of clear vision and allows group members to be aware of all their fellows within the group with a very small movement of the head.

The converse of being able to see everyone else is that everyone can see you, and this makes it very difficult to hide in this group formation. However, it is possible for members to draw back from the group circle as a method of reducing contact with it. Conversely, when they are keenly interested or wish to make a point forcefully they will tend to lean forward. Both these actions may mean something or nothing very much, according to the circumstances in which they occur and to the personalities and behavioural habits of those who employ them. They are traditionally associated with boredom or lack of interest in the first case and with interest and the need to be assertive in the second.

Attention is often given to the positions which members take up within the circle, as defining the kind of role a member wishes to play. But this applies only, if at all, when members have had the opportunity of choosing their position. Thus if each session of a group starts socially, say in one room, and then the members move into another room for the group session and are able to take their seats when all are present, then where they elect to sit may be worthy of some attention.

An aspect of this seating situation often referred to in groupwork literature has been that the person who sits directly opposite the group leader(s) is a potential challenger of that leadership. There is a simple physical explanation for this. In repose the head tends to assume a forward-looking position as this is most comfortable for the neck muscles. In this position the eyes tend to be looking straight forward – that is, they are looking directly at what is opposite. So during the course of a group session the eyes of the leader and the member immediately opposite will tend to be in contact longer than will be the case for other group members. The net result of this may well be that the member sitting opposite the group leader(s) begins to feel either that s/he is under more direct scrutiny than anyone else or that s/he is being offered more cues to contribute to the discussion. Either way s/he is liable to feel mildly uncomfortable and to respond by making a larger and probably more aggressive contribution than s/he would normally have done, either verbally or non-verbally. It must be admitted, however, that when a group member knows this about the position opposite the leader(s) and then deliberately chooses to occupy it, there are some grounds for thinking that this may indeed be the start of a leadership challenge.

If there are two leaders in a group, one of the reasons for their not sitting side by side is that there are then two possible foci of designated leadership power, and this tends to diffuse direct confrontation of this nature.

Although the stress in this book is on being able to see the larger processes which are made up of the small individual and subgroup behaviours, seeing these smaller elements of a group's behaviour is just as important. It is essential to remember that although we may be watching very closely the group's performance as a unit, what group members will take away with them from the group is what they as individuals have been able to learn and experience, and so it is that we also have to keep an eye on what is happening to them as individuals.

Group members frequently find that their experience of being in a group encourages them to risk behaviour which previously they have either avoided, or not suspected lay within their ability to perform. So the idea of personal growth and development has to be monitored. Thus whatever the abilities of members at the beginning of a group, there is the possibility that the group can enhance certain areas. Indeed, this is exactly what a large number of groups are set up to achieve. Equally, of course, the group may have the effect of reducing abilities in some areas and of changing the focus or nature of others. In short, change is a distinct possibility in whatever direction it may lie, and it is essential that the leadership is aware of this.

The more each individual is prepared to put into the group in terms of effort, time and commitment, the more that individual is liable to receive back from the group. This is a very difficult lesson for some people to learn, largely because, for a variety of possible reasons, they find that they cannot allow themselves to trust other people. We are dependent upon others and on being accepted by those whose opinions and respect we value, which sometimes has the effect of producing the fear of 'making a fool of oneself', which has the effect, we feel, of reducing our acceptability in the eyes of others.

This fear and others based upon past experience operate to make people cautious – and under the usual circumstances of our society, quite rightly so. It is interesting to watch a group of strangers meeting for the first time cautiously testing each other out and making assessments based upon previous similar experiences. Some people are so 'closed off' that they can make very few adjustments to new circumstances and are therefore usually disappointed by them. Indeed, their disappointment is often what reaffirms their cautious and suspicious approach.

Now this is a great shame, for a number of reasons, both for those who are 'closed off' and for others with whom they come in contact. It is a fact of group life that when some members hold back their commitment to the group, not only do they reduce what *they* get from the group but they also decrease what is possible for others to get as well. In fact, the degree of commitment that members give to a group, as well as being one of its greatest assets, can be one of its strongest constraints, and the leadership need to be well aware of what is happening in this respect. When commitment is lacking, the effect on the group does not just rest with that lack in, say, an individual member; there is also the effect it has on others. Timid members who are looking for and need strong examples to follow and from which to derive support, may, by a process known as 'contagion', be affected by the closed-off nature of others and produce ultra-cautious behaviour of their own. This is even more so when the closed-off ones are those members who for some reason enjoy high status within the group.

Some of the effects of member status

We have already noted how members of a group tend to take on various operations or roles which eventually become a major part of their life in the group and which other members come to have an expectation that they will perform. Thus one member can usually be relied upon to act as a pacifier in any kind of heated situation which may develop; another seems to keep an eye on the time; another is a reliable spur to getting on with the job; and so on. Most of these roles are beneficial and there is no reason why they should not be exercised by others when they see or feel the necessity of behaving in this way. They are a simple form of a division of labour for the many tasks that most groups need to perform. However, on occasions a role is ascribed to an individual which means that that individual performs it with greater frequency than anyone else and that there has grown an expectation that s/he will act in this way. As long as that member gains satisfaction and a sense of useful participation and is not prevented from doing other things within the group as a result, then no doubt s/he will continue to do so.

However, there are some group roles that occur with great frequency which are of a different nature and need great vigilance by the group leadership in terms of their possible effects. Of these perhaps the most important is one which has come to be called the 'scapegoat'. This role is a frequent headache for groups and leaders, and must be seen to have some very important implications (Douglas, 1995).

There are at least two major forms of scapegoat, temporary and permanent, but there is a great deal of behaviour which is common to both. In the Bible the scapegoat was the animal which was ritually laden with the sins of the community and then driven into the wilderness to die, thus cleansing the people of that particular load of sins. Over time the term has come to be used for those who are blamed not only for their own faults but the faults of others as well. So we find in any community great or small individuals or groups who are blamed when things go wrong, or even when there is a wish that things would go better.

In some senses such individuals and groups draw off much bad feeling, thus freeing the rest of the group to work more productively and harmoniously together. Of course, those who are made scapegoats in this way may not feel that they are conferring any useful benefits on the community of which they are members. They tend to be selected for this role in one of two ways. Either they have an obvious expectation that they will be treated badly and thus draw upon themselves the kind of response they have learned to expect, creating a self-fulfilling prophecy, or they are selected for this role because they demonstrate some very obvious difference from their fellow members. Such differences can be in any area of existence: sex, race, colour, speech, habits, appearance, beliefs, age, intelligence, behaviour, and so on. Difference is a marker. When things are going wrong and there is no obvious rational cause that can be discovered, irrational behaviour tends to take over and blame is allocated to those who are marked in the group by some form of difference. It is usually essential that the scapegoating behaviour does not drive away the elected one but only pushes him/her to the fringes of the group, where s/he remains to be used again if necessary.

Temporary scapegoats tend to occur when the difference which becomes a marker for the others is concerned with that individual's lagging behind when the group is eager to move forward. Such an individual tends to use behaviour patterns which the group as a whole has rejected in favour of newer ones. Because the new patterns are somewhat insecure, when members are reminded of their anxiety about being able to cope with them, they tend to feel dislike for the individual who generates that anxiety, and he/she becomes the target of anger and frustration. When and if the scapegoat's behaviour conforms or s/he leaves the group, the blaming process stops unless the scapegoat was also one of the permanent variety.

The obvious difference of some people seems to incur dislike and a position of being a permanent target. It would appear to be logical that no person would be prepared to tolerate being placed in such a situation, but many do, and we are forced to the conclusion that in some way it provides them with some form of satisfaction.

Example

A young man whose behaviour was quite bizarre on occasions was every week made the focus of some fairly malicious horseplay and ridicule in a therapy group. He continued to attend with unfailing regularity and endured these sessions with good humour. Other members occasionally expressed concern, both at their own behaviour and at the victim's apparent ability to take the ridicule. When he did not come one week they were very concerned and expressed fears that he had been driven away and avowed that they missed him. When he returned, for a short period of time they made a great fuss of him and then gradually reverted to their usual behaviour.

The young man in the group gained more satisfaction from the ridicule of his fellow members than they could credit. He was an isolate, unemployed and could spend whole days without conversing with another being. The attention he received in the group was more than enough of a reward for the ridicule he also received. The group laid off its bad feelings on this one person and was able to work more freely as a result. The eventual outcome was that the group leader created other opportunities for the scapegoat to meet with other people and withdrew him from the group. As a result, for a while the leader accepted the role of scapegoat himself until the group developed other methods of coping with their bad feelings.

The permanent scapegoat tends to be a person who is obviously different from the others but who is also of value to the group and whose level of satisfaction is being met by his/her membership. A very delicate balance is involved here, but even very willing sacrifices are not a good example of leadership and group skills. No one person should be allowed either to make such a sacrifice or be forced into it, for the simple reason that by using this device the group as a whole, including the leader, are evading the task of finding out what is *really* going wrong.

It is well to remember two things in this context:

1   Individuals will tend to stay in situations where the level of their personal satisfaction exceeds their dissatisfaction or when there are no perceived alternatives.
2   Satisfaction in this context is entirely personal and idiosyncratic, often apparently illogical and always complicated by so many factors which are unknown to others that it is always safer to speculate that it exists or that movement is possible than to suppose that it does not, when individuals make no move to change their position.

Feedback

Every day of our lives we make assumptions about other people's behaviour. Where such behaviour tends to fit into the 'normal' patterns that we expect, then the basic assumption that we make is that all is going as usual. Where, in our view, behaviour becomes somewhat odd, we try to work out what sort of reasons could possibly account for it, especially if the people in question are important to us in some way or other. Thus if someone has treated us rather coldly, we may say that they were preoccupied or that therefore they did not notice us. We would probably not be too offended by this. If, however, we thought that the behaviour was occasioned by a deliberate attempt to be offensive, then our reaction could be very different depending on circumstances.

Now if human beings were as logical as they like to think they are, this situation of offence-taking need not arise. The basic assumption about this behavioural event was that it was deliberate and therefore was insulting because that was the intent. Logically, if any element of doubt existed about the intent, then the obvious thing to have done would be to check whether the assumption of intent was correct before acting upon it. Of course, very few people do this, for the simple reason that the feelings engendered by the supposed affront are sufficient to promote retaliation or retreat rather than a request for enlightenment. In any case, few people would feel they have the time to make such requests in the hurly-burly of everyday life.

But this kind of response sours many individual relationships and is often the cause of much unhappiness and misunderstanding. In itself this is bad enough, but when it comes to large organizations which behave in the same way, then the damage can be increased many-fold. This is where the idea of 'feedback' comes in.

Feedback is a term borrowed from cybernetics, where self-regulating mechanisms have been in use for a very long time. Consider the regulator on a steam engine. When the pressure of steam reaches a predetermined level which is regarded as no longer sufficiently safe, it causes a valve to open, allowing the steam to escape until the pressure is reduced to a 'safe' level, when the valve closes. If this principle is applied to human behaviour, then warning has to be given that certain things which are being done at the moment are passing out of the zone of safety. In other words, they are going to cause anger, conflict which is unnecessary, or some other form of hurt. The assumptions which have been made that everything was fine need to be checked out. Feedback implies that some form of information from the system itself is required so that the system can be efficiently regulated. Without that feedback, assumptions about the system's performance may be wholly or partially inaccurate. Any organization can only be as efficient as the feedback it produces and which it then acts upon. Assumptions do not matter a great deal if no action is to be taken on the basis of them. But action based on assumptions which are wrong or out of date, even if done with the best will in the world, can only be as good as those assumptions.

Feedback is important not only in group situations but in all aspects of human relationships, especially where behaviour which can seriously affect the lives of others is going to be based on it. Clearly, it is also one very important way in which we can continuously check on our own self-images, by monitoring the feedback which we get from others about the ways in which they see us behaving, which may be in contrast to the ways in which we think we are performing. In operating with groups it is necessary constantly to monitor the responses of members in order to assure oneself that what is going on is what one thought was going on. It is an essential part of group success that as far as possible all those involved begin to share ideas about the most important elements of the group's existence. This does not mean the eradication of alternative and different ideas. But it does mean that if the group is to exercise its function as an integral unit, then those ideas which relate to the group's essential functions should be held in common by the members. Differences have to be fed into the group and become parts of its growth and developmental patterns, but democratic agreement is fundamental to group progress. Differences need therefore to be known and not hidden as personal agendas which have the effect of reducing the commitment of those members who hold them.

For instance, a member might say, 'What I see happening is that the group appears to be getting involved with things which are not part of its task.' This is a statement of one person's assumption. It is not a statement of absolute fact but a personal comment which in essence is asking for confirmation or otherwise. 'We are not getting on with the task' is an assertion that bears a strong resemblance to a statement of absolute fact and as such does not seek confirmation, but only challenge or agreement. The first statement cannot really be challenged because it is a statement of what one person believes s/he has seen. Other members may have seen something different, and the form of the statement leaves them every opportunity to agree or disagree in the sense that their impressions of what is going on are either similar or dissimilar, a process which should lead to all becoming aware of difference and of being able to reach the areas of consensus. The second statement on the other hand, because it appears to be an absolute and dogmatic assertion of fact, is challengeable. It may be regarded as an authoritative remark by someone who is seen as possessing a great deal of power, in which case it may well be resented by those who disagree, but nevertheless remain unchallenged.

The first statement is, as I have said, a request for confirmation that the way the person who made it sees the situation is the way it is for most of the others. It is asking for feedback, feedback which is necessary in order that actions taken are based upon the situation as it is and not upon some exclusively biased view of it, feedback which is an action, a self-reviewing mechanism which allows any organization or system to take an overall view of what is actually happening and thus to make effective and fact-related decisions about its performance.

TO DECIDE WHAT NEEDS DOING

Of course, the ability to intervene in a group is very dependent upon the observations that have been made of what the group is doing and of what its needs are at any given time. A computer is only as good as the information fed into it, and similarly, intervention in group situations must be based on accurate perceptions of what is happening.

We have seen something of the main ways in which the leadership of a group can operate, but basically they are all redundant if a group is pursuing its ways to its goals with all the skill at its command. Intervention by anyone, leader or not, can be justified on only two grounds. The first of these is personal, i.e. to save oneself or others from some real or perceived danger, and the second, to attempt to move the group more into line with achieving the goals which it has set for itself when there is evidence that it has deviated from that course. Now in the case of the leader of a newly formed group there will often be little ability on the part of most of the other members either to see what is needed or to be able to know what to do about it even if they are perceptive enough to see that something needs to be done. Thus the responsibility falls on the leadership to make such moves as are necessary. This redresses what was going awry or sets in motion events which were not being initiated. If this is done with skill and perception, it will also have shown members the way in which some future interventions can be made by them and perhaps given them some idea of their potential power to use the group for their avowed ends. This means that the original intervention has to be achieved without making it appear that such events can be achieved only by those with an enormous amount of skill and experience to back it up. This is usually done by revealing the thinking and observational processes that went into making such an intervention. Of course, if the group leadership want the group to be dependent upon their skill and knowledge all the time, then no such concession needs to be made, for it is not part of the group contract that the members should be helped to increase their group skills.

Intervention must have a focus. That is, it must be used in an area of group behaviour which is important to either group achievement or group survival. To be able to be focused means that the group leadership must be clearly aware of the purposes of the group and also equally clear about whether what is going on at the moment is leading towards or away from those purposes.

Example

A group were discussing their progress after several months of work. What the leader could see quite clearly was that collectively the group believed that they had failed, and almost unanimously attributed that failure to their own level of competence, so much so that they obliterated much consideration of any other possible causative factors. The leader very gradually insinuated into their discussion several elements of the complex inter-organizational situation in which they worked, pointing out that they had not set the parameters which limited time with clients; rather, the judicial system had. It was the leader's intention to direct their discussion not to their own defects as groupworkers but to the design of the group system in which they operated and to try to assess where changes could be made in their programme which would most probably ensure that their efforts produced a much better level of success.

It is significant that the intervention recorded here not only dealt with the immediate needs of the depressed members but was also vitally concerned with the survival of the group. What eventually ensued was a successful attempt to redesign the programme, given that they had now a much better understanding of the effects of the constraints imposed upon them by the external system of which they were a part.

Initiation ceremonies

The illustration below is taken from my records of a group of patients discharged from psychiatric care when they had been meeting as a group for several months. During the existence of the group no new member had been added. The illustration is a good example not only of an initiation ceremony but also of the problems which often face a newcomer to an established group and of the expectations people have of such situations.

Example

At the request of the psychiatrist, another person was to join the group. Preparations were duly made in that the admission of the new member was discussed with the group and his suitability for membership ascertained. The new member was informed of the group's progress to date and what the general norms of behaviour were. He was then introduced to the group and for several weeks the established members were kindness itself to him. Then there was a noticeable cooling in their attitudes, though they were always polite. The leader could find no obvious reason for this and could get no response from the members either by direct questioning about it or by hinting that he would like to know what was wrong. Eventually, one of the members, in the course of a discussion with the leader on an entirely different topic, muttered something like, 'Well, he hasn't talked, you know . . . he hasn't said a thing . . .' It dawned on the leader that he had forgotten that the group had established in its early stages a norm of 'confession' as the price of acceptance. The 'new' member was discreetly informed of this and at

97

the next session he began his contribution by saying, 'I think I ought to tell you about myself.' He was listened to in interested silence and then the questions began.

From that moment on he was a full member of the group with access to all their secrets and counsels. Needless to say, the leader made a point of bringing out into the open the initiation rite which had occurred and also of suggesting to the group that in future they might try helping people to see what was required of them.

This kind of situation is very common. In fact, some group leaders make a point of using such ceremonies to emphasize that something is happening, to draw attention to it, and so make members aware of what is going on. It is important to recognize that anyone tends to be most vulnerable when in transition from a state of security or familiarity to one of uncertainty. The whole problem of the 'new' member is of this order.

Another point which this example shows clearly is the difference between an open group and a closed one.

Open and closed groups

In the simplest possible definition, open groups are those which never close their doors to the admission of new members. This means that they are constantly having to be concerned with the problem of the 'newcomer'. Members leave and members are added, so the problem of saying goodbye to someone who has worked with you for a period of time and hello to new and unknown members occurs fairly frequently.

Because of the changes in members, such groups never seem to develop the intense relationships which are usually found in closed groups. They also have some difficulties in maintaining a sufficient number of members at any one time to act as the 'core' of the group, which has the responsibility of transmitting the group's peculiar culture – that is, the norms and standards and values which that group has developed over the period of its existence. In this sense the nature of the group, i.e. whether it is open or closed, can be seen as a constraint, but not one that is insurmountable. In fact, the very nature of the difference can be used in order to achieve certain outcomes.

Individuals who have found some difficulty in making and breaking relationships will be able to get much more practice in how this can be done effectively in a group which is open rather than in one which is closed and thus sheltered from the hassle of newcomers and leavers. Likewise, individuals who need the support of a few ongoing relationships so that they are able to develop the ability to trust others will be much better served in a group which has a static membership. Recognizing that the open or closed nature of a group creates peculiar possibilities means quite simply that such possibilities should be taken into consideration right from the planning stage of the group and not discovered as problems halfway through the group's life.

ASSESSING THE EFFECT OF WHAT HAS BEEN DONE

Recording

Making a detailed record of what a group has been doing has always been a very sore point with groupworkers for a variety of reasons. It seems to have been consistently regarded as a form of drudgery with nothing like the excitement of actually working with a group. *But it is absolutely essential and must not be ignored.* The ability that any one person may have to keep track of the interactions of several people, especially when involved in the same process which s/he is trying to recall, is at best extremely limited. At worst it is disastrously biased and very selective.

As we have seen, the efficiency of a group's leadership will depend to a large extent on the ability to make critical judgements based on an understanding of the situation in the group. Given that it is relatively easy to pay attention to the interactions between individuals and subgroups as they occur, it is much less easy to see how these small interactions add up to large movements in the group's life without some form of recording which can be examined at leisure and free from the obligations of being a leader.

Again the only way in which a leader can be in any way sure that s/he has the situation clear is for that leader to have been making continuous assessments of the progress which the group has made. This means seeing the large movements of the group, which are the processes that, as we have seen, are made up of the small and more immediate movements in the group.

This has to be done over a period of time, for it takes time for the small activities to aggregate into the larger ones. But if the activities of the group have not been recorded in some way which allows access to a continuous record, the group leadership has only memory rather than knowledge on which to plan work with the group. So much tends to intervene between one group session and another that memory alone is extremely fallible. In one particular way it tends to be more fallible than in others, and that is in recalling sequence. The processes grow out of an accretion of smaller events, but it is the order in which the smaller events occurred which will, more than anything, dictate the intensity and quality of the process which emerges. That order is something that without recording tends to be remembered in terms of what was most important to the specific individual doing the recalling and not to the overall group.

The process of working with a group may be very involved and subject to vexations and sweat-producing problems. But this is no reason for ignoring one instrument which is as essential as the original design and planning. It is logical to realize that some form of recording is necessary. The muddle and confusion can only be made worse if an unsystematic approach is used. There is no substitute for the practice of 'recall in tranquillity' – that is, to sit down and record what has gone on immediately a group has finished, using whatever notes have been made during the course of the group. Of course, there are the group members who can be consulted, there are co-leaders and any other observers. Any tactic which will obviate bias and add to the available store of information and sequence may be used.

Failure to recognize what has happened

It is not always easy to recognize and assess what has happened in a group, or to know what the appropriate responses may be. In an article written as long ago as 1968, Kenneth Heap told the following apposite story of a group-worker's failure to recognize the signs of change in her group.

Example

The worker had set up a group which was a social club specifically to cater for the needs of elderly men who were becoming increasingly isolated. She proceeded to meet each of the men she felt might benefit from such a club and established a good working relationship with each of them. She used this relationship, which she described as 'they made me feel like a loved, but managing daughter', to try to generate good interaction amongst the group members, and she herself operated as the group leader. As the men found common purpose and became identified with the club they began also to take over the running of it. After some months the worker had not noticed that their dependency upon her had changed until one day the members approached her. With some guilt and discomfort they asked whether she had not more important things she could be doing than spending an evening every week with them. They assured her that they would quite understand if she wanted to leave and get on with something else.

This is a very clear indication of the need of a group's leadership to keep abreast of developments within the group. It is also a good illustration of the responsibility that comes to the person who decides to create a group to meet some kind of perceived need. It cannot be stressed too often that once a group so created begins to function, then the need that brought it into existence has, almost without question, changed, and the style of leadership which originated with the group may well need to change also.

Stage-by-stage example

Stage 3: Operation

As an essential part of the basic contract had been that the group would use itself as a model for learning about group processes in general, this was now put into effect. It had also been accepted that any increase in personal awareness which resulted from this would be a bonus, but such was not the primary objective. This point is crucial. It is quite easy for an element of deceit to emerge here. Many groups which have been started for purposes other than exploring self-awareness seem to have turned into exactly such groups. Now, this is unfair and unethical for any number of reasons. Several of the members of such a group might well not have contracted to become members of it had they known at the time that it would develop in this unscheduled way. Once in a group, it is often somewhat difficult to get out because of the group pressures and the sense of probably letting other people down. Such members have thus had a very good lesson in being conned, and whatever level of trust they may have started to develop in groupwork will certainly be stunted, if not killed off, by this kind of treatment.

I do not think it necessary to detail the day-by-day operation of this group. Suffice it to say that the principal acts of leadership were divided into three substages:

1 Most effort in the early stages was put into the slow transfer from didactic teaching and information-giving to experiential learning. Although a large amount of information was still being conveyed, it was now made relevant to what was actually happening in the group at the time. When the group were trying to decide whether the behaviour of one member was appropriate and conformed to the aims of the group, the informational input was related to the ways in which groups establish norms and standards of behaviour. When yet another member was being challenged for appearing to want to take over the group, the input related to concepts of social power and to acts of leadership.

2 In the middle period, the efforts were divided between maintaining the group as an entity over the various breaks which occurred (vacations, etc.) and encouraging the members to make their own inputs based upon their own experience and learning. As a member would start to explain what s/he saw as happening in the group, other members were encouraged to offer their contributions so that the

originally centrally focused group started to become much more openly reliant on all its resources rather than on just one.

3   The third period was characterized by a great reduction of leadership acts on my part, especially those of a controlling nature, and an increase in 'working' acts. This meant that at different times different members of the group took control of the group and my 'talking' contributions rapidly diminished. The analysis of what was happening to the group then depended upon some member of the group feeling moved to deliver his/her observations and to run with the responses s/he received. This was also the time when the sense of accountability of each of the group's members, not just for themselves but for the group as a whole, increased quite dramatically.

During this period the group drew much closer together and started to spend some of their spare time in each other's company. They began to feel that they were a unit, and opposition from other areas of the course tended to reinforce this feeling. I set tasks for them to be performed outside the group sessions which could have been achieved in any of several ways. They chose to do them as a group and to submit their results as a unit, each member standing or falling on the quality of their united work.

The insights into the ways in which they worked as a group came fairly thick and fast at this time. A great problem was how to find the time for them to be able to relate what was happening in their group to their knowledge of what happened in groups generally. The pressures outside the group continued to exert influence and the level of trust did not develop beyond a level which was appropriate to facilitate their learning. The personal growth bonus was thus quite small, and certainly different for different individuals. Relationships became more open and some friendships blossomed mildly. I was more and more treated as someone who could be trusted, and the level of warmth in the group grew.

The problem of the course assessment was solved by being made upon the performance of the group as a whole, consonant with the group's choice to work as a unit when given the opportunity. After all, the purpose of the group was to learn about group processes, and this could just as well be measured in terms of the group's performance as a whole as of that of individual members.

8

WHERE RESPONSIBILITY LIES

However a group is actually run, whether by directive leadership, by mutual consent or other method, there is no escaping the fact that those who call the group into existence in the first place continue to have some responsibility for its maintenance unless and until that responsibility has been seen to be transferred to some elected or chosen member or members. And to that end we must consider those acts which when made in the group are intended to move the group in some direction or other, or bring the members to consider what they are doing, where they are going and whether they are on course to achieve what they set out to do.

This brings into question all the various facts about leadership, which is indeed a very vexed subject. This is not the place to go into the many theories and ideas which have been circulated about it, and which can be read about in the literature on groupwork. What I want to suggest is that it is preferable to leave the whole question of leadership in favour of a look at what might be called 'leadership acts', for the simple reason that in any group, and in some groups much more than others, it is not only the 'designated' leader or natural leader who will make moves to shift the group in a given direction; so will many other members. Indeed, the only qualifications needed for making this kind of move are that a member can see that some kind of move is necessary, that the member feels that s/he has some kind of idea about what is required, and, very importantly, that it is worth taking the risk to offer it.

In essence we are talking about behaviours deployed by group members which are designed, or which at least have as their basic motivation, the perceived need to move the group in one direction or another. Because these moves can be made by any member we can look at the nature of such acts and how they work more or less independently of who makes them.

Much has already been said about the need for leadership and the problems which underlie its acceptance in current Western society. Basically it is a question of the exercise of power, and as there is a very strong current running at the moment which favours the development of the use of power strategies in those who obviously have been prevented, or who were unable, to use them in the past, the concept of leadership acts is essentially compatible

103

with that thesis. Leadership acts which move any group towards the achievement of its avowed goals are to be encouraged, and those which hinder or obstruct the achievement of such goals are to be discouraged. The problem is not to decide who shall make such moves, as all groupworkers discover, but to become able to decide which is which, to be able to recognize good moves when they occur. They do not always advertise their presence upon first appearance, or indicate clearly what their eventual consequences will be.

This is what I meant when suggesting, in the title of this chapter, that responsibility lies with whoever takes on the business of trying to move the group in any way whatsoever, whoever they may be.

One of the main problems with regard to making leadership acts is concerned with what the helping professions sometimes call 'the conscious use of self'. This rather elaborate phrase seems to mean that in working with people it is necessary to be aware that the 'instrument' with which one is working is oneself. There are habitual behaviours which have to be set aside and customary responses which have to be monitored for the effects that they produce, in pursuit of, for instance, the aim of not dominating when what the group requires is the encouragement to express ideas and feelings of its own. Most individuals who willingly take on the role of group leader will most probably be quite determined and forceful persons with good verbalizing skills, a very useful asset in verbally oriented Western societies. But the use of such skills can intrude too much into the group situation and preclude the participation of other members who have nothing like the same verbal ability, or, in many cases, the knack of being able to create space for their ideas to be heard.

There is a distinct difference between the behaviours which are appropriate to managing a group and the habitual behaviours of everyday existence. There is also a distinct difference between knowing about this and being able to do it in practice. Making leadership acts, whoever makes them, requires a skill which can be learned.

LEADERSHIP ACTS

For convenience in explanation, leadership acts can be divided into three categories:

1 *Working moves*. These are basically concerned with keeping the group as a functioning unit and may be concerned either with the task which the group is trying to achieve or with the relationships between the members.
2 *Control moves*. These are acts which are concerned more explicitly with bringing about changes in the group's behaviour patterns, for instance by encouraging behaviours which a member or a leader can see are taking

the group towards what it is trying to achieve and, alternatively, trying to stop or reduce those acts which are seen as preventing the group from doing this.

3   *Self-preservation moves.* This is a self-evident category of acts, which are often leadership acts only in that they are attempts to head off group behaviours which an individual believes, rightly or wrongly, to be threatening. It is frequently discovered that such moves set a precedent for other members equally feeling threatened, and thus they can and do alter the behaviour patterns of the group.

Let us look at these moves in more detail.

Working moves

The difference between task and relationship leadership acts is widely covered in the literature and is, in fact, often referred to there as a clear distinction between kinds of leadership.

No group which requires even minimal co-operation for the achievement of its goals will actually work together if it has not spent some time and effort in establishing the appropriate degree of safety for its members to do so. If members are directing a considerable amount of their energy to the purpose of maintaining their own safety, then that same energy cannot also be directed to working at the group's job. When members join a group, most often they are entering a situation which possesses sufficient strangeness to promote a level of anxiety which may well be inhibiting of commitment. This is perfectly normal behaviour and is equally well observed when an individual enters a new job with new colleagues. He/she does not know the ropes and moves with some degree of caution until some of those ropes become apparent. Group literature refers to this as the development of an appropriate level of trust. In this case 'appropriate' means a level at which a reasonable degree of energy can be committed to the group task.

Example

A group of students whose main task was to use their own group in order to learn some of the ubiquitous facts about groups found that they were unable to proceed beyond the point of discussing the structure of their group. Time after time, with the best intentions in the world they could only try to establish the rules under which they were prepared to proceed to the main task. Even this eluded them; they could not even agree about the way in which they would proceed. Eventually, after many weeks of this kind of procedure, one member ventured to say that he was unable to be open about what he wanted the group to achieve because he was awed by the experience and qualifications of other members of the group, which he perceived as far exceeding his own. Once this point was out into the open it became evident that several other members of the group had similar feelings of inferiority which had made them very cautious. Now the problem could be discussed and dealt with.

Intervention

However much we may try to evade this issue by using different terms, we have to face the fact that groupwork is an interventive and manipulative procedure. Whichever way we proceed in working with a group, there is always the implication that it is set up to benefit its members and others, and in that sense we are talking about change and/or support.

The continuum of leadership acts goes from controlling and directive behaviour at one end to enabling, guiding and facilitating at the other. But at whichever end of this continuum any one person operates, or whether s/he moves to different parts of the scale of leadership acts as opportunity and need allow, the process is still one of attempting to bring about some kind of change. The very presence of an acknowledged leader within a group affects the behaviour of others in a way that depends on their perception of the leader and what s/he can do. Equally, the presence of individual members affects the kind of behaviour the leader(s) will deploy. Whatever knowledge and understanding of group process and of human behaviour a member possesses will be the source of that member's actions and thinking in the group even if s/he feels compelled to withhold what in other circumstances s/he would normally have offered. Individual behaviour in a group is selective in the sense that what is offered is only a part of the behavioural repertoire available.

If leadership is recognized not so much as a specialized function, the sole perquisite of one or two designated persons, but as residing in acts which any member of the group may make, then the designated leaders will initially be the ones who make more leadership acts than others, because of their greater expertise and knowledge in the specific area of groupwork. If and when other members develop groupworking skills, then the number of leadership acts designated leaders may make will tend to decrease. But the timing of this decrease has to be appropriate to the level of readiness of others. It has always seemed to me to be totally unethical for any leader to unload his/her responsibilities for the group onto members who, by the very nature of the exercise, must be less aware of what is involved than the leader. Such transfer of power and responsibility needs to be part of a well-thought-out scheme to introduce members to the art of leadership and based upon a clear perception that the members are capable of coping. Let me give an example of what this means.

A group leader may say to his members at the beginning of some group exercises that they have a clear right not to take part in what is about to happen, if that is what they want. This can be seen as an indication of the leader's understanding of the natural reluctance of the members to enter into something which may be unfamiliar and about which they have some misgivings. The responsibility to join or not to join has been handed to the individual members. But there are other considerations which are not so obvious. On what basis can such a choice be made? Without experience and knowledge of such exercises, there is little logical basis for choice. Can the choice be made on emotional grounds? Well yes, it can. But how does a leader know what those grounds might be? It is not possible to know totally what pressures brought individuals to the group in the first place or what pressures are keeping them there now. If one member feels s/he would like to opt out, how far is that behaviour going to be influenced by perceptions of the kind of response such an act will elicit from the others? And how much does it matter?

It is known that the expectations individuals have of a situation are created by a complex of factors, and straight information of apparent intent is interpreted in the light of this complex. It is the responsibility of every group leader to contain the responsibility for decisions within him/herself until such time as they can be shared with the group members and used to start the process of enhancing their understanding of the complex nature of the pressures involved as a basis for their becoming able to exercise responsibility for the group in their own right.

By taking on the role of group leader, by convening a group, by taking over an existing group, a leader has already intervened in the lives of others to some extent and as a result must be aware of the need to accept responsibility for the consequences of those actions. It is of no consequence that the leader's intentions were of a benign nature; the conscious act of intervention, a deliberate interference in the lives of others, whether at their request or as part of a statutory obligation or based upon some idea of conferring benefit, entails responsibility for the consequences. A chain of actions has been set in motion that would not have occurred in that form, or perhaps at all, without the conscious intent of the instigator.

In many areas of everyday life this sequence is of little consequence because, rightly or wrongly, we assume that sufficient knowledge exists on the part of those involved to make their involvement or otherwise a conscious and informed choice. After all, the basic skill of the cheat is to ensure that his/her victims believe that they have sufficient information on which to base a logical and conscious choice, when s/he knows in fact that they have not. But few people can be held to possess even a limited understanding of the complex processes of human interaction. Those who work professionally have an obligation for that understanding to be of a better order of sophistication than the general level.

There are thus two active possibilities and one passive one. Let us consider the third first. If, possessing some knowledge of group behaviour, the leader has no intention of using it either for or against the interests of others, then the ethical considerations are of little interest. Of the two remaining possibilities, one is to assume a paternalistic attitude of superior wisdom and to apply one's knowledge and skill, like a doctor, apparently for the benefit of others, without making any attempt to enhance their understanding of what is involved. The other is to apply one's knowledge directly to the matters involved and also to the development of an increased understanding of what is happening so that the others in the situation can begin to appreciate the process. This leads to their being able to make choices based upon understanding, and to being able to assume a real responsibility for themselves and not one which may be based upon ignorance or half-truth.

In the light of this, we can now look at the process of intervention in a group situation, bearing in mind that either of the two processes may be involved, or even a continuum from one to the other as circumstances change. It would tend to follow from what has been said so far that intervention comprises leadership acts and that these are not necessarily the prerogative of any designated leader. It should be helpful to isolate for scrutiny four different categories of leadership acts:

- acts which seek to smooth relationships and establish and maintain the possibility of group members working together;
- acts which are deliberately initiated to move the group towards the achievement of any tasks it may have;
- acts which deliberately exercise control over the whole group process, are directive and tend to be long-sighted and goal-directed;
- acts which are concerned with personal survival and are usually initiated by one member to enhance personal security.

Before we look at these leadership acts in some detail, it must be remembered that intervention is usually deployed in order to change something which is happening. But there are exceptions, for example when what is occurring in the group is fine and intervention is made to stop change taking place and to ensure a continuation of what is already going on.

The number of ways of achieving change is actually quite small. Member behaviour can be enhanced – that is, encouraged; diminished – that is, reduced; changed to something else by the introduction of some new factors; or eliminated by a total change to new factors. These changes can be directed in different ways. For instance, one member may be making all the running and, in the process, moving the group further and further away from its basic objectives and using up scarce and valued time. Intervention to bring about change could be directed at the individual by diminishing, eliminating or redirecting his/her contribution; by encouraging contributions from other members; by bringing in other factors from outside the group; and so on. In short, intervention can be directed at individuals, subgroups, the total group and key external factors.

Smoothing relationships

It must be apparent from what has been said so far that in modern society working together happily does not occur easily. People are suspicious of strangers and even of loved ones. Individuals have some degree of anxiety that they will appear to others in a manner which is different from the way in which they would like to be seen. We all maintain a public façade, a presentation of ourselves which we believe to be acceptable. It is not surprising therefore that in any collection of individuals, particularly of strangers, energy is devoted by everyone to ensuring that they are safe by using techniques refined by past experience which have been relatively successful. Equally unsurprisingly, until some degree of security, usually associated with growing familiarity, has been established, the amount of energy available for working together is diminished by the amount devoted to security in the form of defence.

Example

In a prison, a group of women was formed of those who had long-term sentences. The objective was to facilitate the exchange of information about the ways in which the long spell of incarceration could be coped with. The group appeared keen and enthusiastic and enjoyed the weekly sessions, but never seemed able to tackle the task which had been contracted at the beginning of the group, despite urging by the group leader. Gradually it emerged that the group leader had assumed that, being part of a small prison system, the women would all know one another well and that well- developed relationships would exist between people with a common bond. This proved to be almost the reverse of the fact, as the women's relationships were limited to pairings and they were, if anything, more suspicious of each other than they were of the leader, who was a probation officer. When they recognized this fact they were able to establish working relationships which enabled them to address their task and to reduce their need to protect themselves.

Because this occurred in a situation in which there were many constraints operating against the development of appropriate trust between the group members and between them and the group leader, the latter had to use a technique of selective reinforcement. Thus as behaviour appeared which seemed to indicate the beginning of trust in either of these two major areas, the leader encouraged it, making sure that the behaviour was made explicit and any warm feelings attached to it made known to all. The leader also offered her personal behaviour as a role model of the kind of norms which she believed would facilitate the development of working relationships. As a representative of authority she was the obvious target of suspicion, and was accused of being a spy, even if a friendly one, or some kind of researcher. Where experience and knowledge cannot provide credible answers to the kind of questions the women in the group were initially asking, then fantasy will tend to fill the gap, and the nature of that fantasy is dependent upon the individual's perceptions of the situation.

Elsewhere in this book emphasis has been laid upon the fact that a collection of people gathered together at the same time and occupying the same space does not necessarily constitute a group in the sense of being a unit with a sense of belonging and of identity. Much work needs to be done to establish working relationships to turn that collection into a 'group', which will free energy to devote to the task in hand.

Getting on with the job

There is no specific point at which it is possible to say that before it a group did not work as a unit and that after it it did. At least, that is my experience. What tends to happen is that at any time the collection of people is able to achieve something but what can be done is always dependent upon the nature of the job they are together to do and how well they have developed the appropriate skills of working together. The more threatening the task, the more co-operation is required, and the more commitment to the group – and the less likely a group is to make much progress with that task in the early stages of its existence. This does not and should not ever prevent a leader from encouraging behaviour which s/he sees as task-oriented, unless it is also obvious that such behaviour has the possibility of being counter-productive in the sphere of relationships.

In a committee, which is a group with a very clearly defined structure, it is always noticeable that members can work quite well together provided that the matters under consideration have little or no strong emotional relevance in a personal way to any member present. The structure creates the parameters inside which it is possible to work without the development of close personal relationships. When issues arise which do concern members personally, then the structure has to be reinforced, and often even then cannot contain the emotions that may be aroused. Because a committee is a special kind of group, it is a collection of individuals bound by a set of rules which are agreed as a condition of membership. There is not often the degree of trust present which would be able to contain such emotions and permit their expression and working through in a climate of safety.

Task-oriented leadership acts are concerned with getting on with the job in hand. Some members are more aware than others of those matters which impinge upon job completion, probably due to personality factors – that is, they are habitually concerned to finish what they start. Some members are usually very conscious of the fact that time is slipping away, that the group is in need of further information, advice, help, etc.; of the need for checking on what has been achieved so far; of the need to encourage others to produce ideas and to discuss them; to perform tasks relevant to the group's overall aim; and so on. When these perceptions are verbalized, they contribute towards getting the job done. They are guides, nudges, indicators of loss of direction or of impetus, and are valuable in restoring and redirecting the group's energy into the way of achievement.

Either of the two categories of leadership act discussed here can be performed by any member of a group who has the perception to see what s/he believes is needed. In groups where members have little or no group experience, however, such acts must fall to the leader, who should initiate them and also encourage others to follow suit to develop the ability of members to become aware of their responsibility for the group's governance and business.

Example

A group of church members had gathered to make a decision about joint services with a neighbouring church. The minister very carefully opened the meeting by explaining what was involved. He also pointed out that a decision had to be made at this meeting in order that it could be passed to the neighbouring church committee in a few days' time. As the members felt strongly about the issue, the discussion was at times heated and reiterative. The minister drew his members back to the task by summing up what had been said for and against and by asking whether everyone was prepared to take a vote on the matter. Towards the end of the meeting he began intimating that time was running out. The committee members eventually faced the necessity of making a decision, realizing that they had exhausted most of the arguments, and voted on the issue.

The exercise of control

Almost inevitably, the acts which come within the 'exercise of control' category are those of a skilled, knowledgeable and experienced group leader. Control implies that its exercise should be based upon a very wide understanding of a group's existence, a view which is comprehensive enough to be aware of the current situation and to be able to see it in the context of what it might develop into. Thus control implies being able to assess which of the

111

group's larger processes will be valuable to it, which may be detrimental and which may be of little or no significance. The kind of long-sighted view necessary to make this kind of assessment comes only from experience of trying and failing and of trying and succeeding. It is rarely the kind of ability found in individuals without experience and training, though in some areas of group life some individuals seem to have an instinctive knowledge of which processes should be encouraged and which should not.

With every new group, a skilled leader is faced with a whole series of complex possibilities. Until s/he has tested and tried some of them s/he cannot regard areas of this complex as known. Gradually s/he can begin to recognize response patterns and the shapes of behaviour. S/he becomes increasingly able to predict with some degree of accuracy what the long-term outcomes will most likely be. At this stage s/he can, if necessary, try to moderate the behaviour of the group to facilitate the development of those patterns which s/he believes will best serve the ends of the group.

For example, a group leader may well find that the totally inexperienced members expect that everything that happens within the group will stem from the leader. But the purpose of the group could be that the members should learn to be aware of the group's processes so that they can choose what they would like to do with them. In short, the leader's aim in this case is to move the group to becoming more self-directing. In order to change the dependency set of such members, the leader will need to take a long-term view of what processes will best meet this end. Paradoxically, s/he may choose to exert such overall control that this control will be eventually recognized for what it is. Then that recognition will become part of their learning process and the control of the leader can be adapted and decreased as the members' learning becomes activated.

The processes which were identified in Chapter 4 are usually the focus of any attempts at control. This is because the processes are fundamental to the group and they are large, as opposed to the relatively small patterns of immediate interaction, and therefore to influence them implies having a larger and more permanent effect.

Basically, a group leader has at his/her command a series of possible intervention techniques which will be used as judgement directs, bearing in mind the capabilities of the group, its level of development and the aims it has set. It may seem trite to say this, but in all simplicity, the techniques are mainly concerned with keeping going things which are effective; stopping behaviours which are destructive; reducing those which are not helpful or changing them to something more useful by a process of redirection; and finally, initiating and encouraging the development and continuation of positively beneficial acts. This is much easier to write about than it is to do, for in practice such actions can be complicated by the possibility of wrong assessment of the value of current behaviour patterns, and second, by the choice of mode of intervention.

Example

After several sessions the group had begun to gel. 'I feel that I can tell you about the fears I had on joining this group,' said one member. The group leader felt that this was a move in the right direction and encouraged the member to speak out. The encouragement was too positive; the member became embarrassed at becoming the centre of attention when in fact she had been speaking her thoughts out loud, and dried up.

The leader's assessment had been accurate as far as it went but had missed the nuances of the personal situation. However, all was not lost. The leader recorded in his mind that a breakthrough in group trust could not be very far away and he needed to remain very alert.

The stimulation or retardation of processes can be achieved in several ways, and sometimes by a combination of efforts. The desired movement may be achieved by attempting to modify the behaviour of an individual member whose current standing in the group is great, or that of a subgroup, or that of the group as a whole. It may also sometimes be done by involving factors from outside the group.

In the example given above, the leader was attempting to encourage the behaviour of an individual which was clearly leading towards what he felt was desirable. It is always risky to do this with one member, especially in the early days of a group, as that person may well be out of step with the rest of the group and thus gain no support from them when set up as a pacemaker.

Sometimes individuals seek support from fellow members, and when they get it a 'pairing' is born. If the pairing becomes an established fact, then a subgroup is being formed and other members may join it or oppose it at different times. Some experts maintain that most of the strongest bids for change in a group come from powerful subgroups. I would agree that this is usually so, and it is important that a group leader should be aware of this process so that s/he can use his/her influence to attempt to influence the behaviour of such subgroups for the benefit of the group as a whole in much the same way as s/he would with a key individual.

Example

A group were discussing what were acceptable methods of making personal comments about fellow members. John had made a remark about Betty which Tim had found unacceptable and had said so. Betty admitted that she had not minded Tim's comment, which had been along the lines that he thought she sounded uninterested in the group's business, saying that she had been thinking much the same herself although she was not really uninterested. Other members said that they had not gained the impression that Betty was upset by what John had said. Betty agreed. The group leader, realizing that here was an opening to try to form a working rule concerning personal comment within his particular group, took the comments of the members and suggested that they seemed to be agreeing that if such comments were made in the way John had made his – that is, sensitively – they were fine. Sally and Chris then picked up on this and said that as long as the comments were an honest reflection of what one saw, they were acceptable, at least as a basis for discussion.

A fundamental rule of procedure had been established.

The group leader here was encouraging Sally and Chris in their explanation of what was an acceptable method of making personal comment. In terms of processes he was attempting to establish a norm of behaviour by enhancing and encouraging the contribution of the small subgroup of Sally and Chris, having decided that Betty, who had been the focus of the interchange, was more than halfway inclined to agree with the conclusions of the subgroup. Interestingly enough, information was being fed in at a point where it was most relevant, i.e. that personal comments can be made in hurtful or in constructive ways – the latter usually by referring to what one person perceives rather than by making a bald statement that something *is*. Perceptions can be inaccurate; statements have an element of challenge. Thus, 'You are behaving in an irresponsible way' is a challenge, however true it may be, and will no doubt tend to provoke a defence which, unless challenge was what was intended, is not the best possible way to promote a possible change in the observed behaviour. By contrast, to say that the behaviour appears to you to be irresponsible is a statement of what you believe you have seen and what you feel, and is usually seen as a personal statement and less challenging. When relationships are well developed in a group, direct challenges are quite acceptable, but by then the mechanisms for dealing with the possible ensuing conflict to the benefit of all concerned will in all probability exist.

The possible range of leadership acts which are controlling in nature can be displayed as follows:

Acts of control achieved by:	on the behaviour of:	to modify one or more of the group processes:
1 stopping	1 individuals	1 interaction
2 reducing	2 subgroups	2 development
3 keeping going	3 total group	3 structure
4 encouraging	4 external factors	4 subgroup formation
5 changing the focus of	5 a combination of two or more of the above	5 goal formation
		6 decision-making
		7 norms, standards and values
		8 cohesion
		9 influence
		10 climate

and requires foresight and an accurate assessment of the value of the behaviour involved in achieving the long-term interests of the group.

Often processes will be affected by drawing the attention of the total group to what is happening, discussing whether this is what the group wants to happen, and if not, seeking for and suggesting ways to bring about change. For instance, the leader can draw attention to the fact that the climate of the group is changing, becoming flat say, with enthusiasm dying away. This is not the responsibility of any single member, and it must therefore be brought to the consideration of the whole group and, if possible, a change created in a way that is beneficial and supportive of the group's purpose.

No group exists in isolation. It is affected by the environment in which it exists, and in turn supplies some stimulus to that milieu. As we have seen, the members bring feelings, beliefs, desires and behaviour patterns into the group and they take out with them attitudes and understandings which they have developed within it. It stands to reason therefore that another way of affecting the processes within a group involves the intervention of outside elements.

Example

A group had been formed by a social worker for the purpose of introducing some local parents to the idea of becoming foster parents. As the group had been founded on the basis of *interest*, one female member was discovered to have had considerable experience in the past of fostering, whereas none of the other members had any at all. This one woman dominated the group's proceedings and could not be dissuaded. As a result, the group was beginning to fall apart because of the members' uncertainty and divided loyalty. The social worker discussed the problem with her superiors, and the experienced foster parent was withdrawn from the group on the basis that she would be more valuable in another context.

Here we have an example of the use of outside elements, in this case the social worker's seniors, in order that the remaining group members were not overwhelmed and were able to establish the group at the level appropriate to their needs. It was unfortunate that the personality of the experienced parent made it too risky to attempt to involve her in a positive way by using her experience. But it did become possible to use her in another group where most of the members were as experienced as she.

Leadership acts which exercise some degree of control over a group like these can eventually be used by any member of a group once the necessary understanding and assessment skills have developed. There are two points to be made about this:

- Directive leadership should not be avoided on the grounds that it is reprehensible to attempt to control others. Such leadership may be an essential first step in the empowerment of members to control the group themselves, or in enabling the group to survive in difficult times.
- Leadership acts require some degree of skill and understanding, and it takes time to acquire them, time which can often be obtained only during a period of security when someone else is monitoring and controlling the overall situation.

Loss of control and self-preservation

Personal security can make life very complicated for the beginning groupworker. Whatever role such an individual takes, whatever his/her aim, one thing is inevitably true, which is that s/he tends to be on his/her own until such time as the group accepts him/her for whatever value they perceive s/he has. Numerically the leader(s) is in a minority even when co-leadership is employed. This is especially true in the time before the group has gelled into a working unit, when the expectations members may have of the leadership's performance are speculative and to a large extent based upon their own desires rather than upon reality.

How often do groupworkers find themselves in the situation of being expected to be experts, omniscient beings on whom group members feel they are going to be able to rely utterly, when the leadership's own feelings of their competence have not actually been very high? Alternatively, group members, especially those who find themselves in groups they have no wish to be in, can be aggressive, challenging and destructive, having expectations which are almost wholly negative.

Such situations and others like them tend to be due to the fact that strange situations and unfamiliarity with what is expected engender anxiety. Responses to this vary enormously, usually on the basis of past experience and habitual preferences. For example, one response might be that of over-whelming expectation of support from one whose status is enhanced out of all proportion in order to assure oneself of the great security such a figure can offer. Another might be aggressive behaviour, which can serve to mask fears and underlying insecurity.

The more anxious a leader may be about his/her own shortcomings, about his/her performance and ability, the more his/her attention and energy will tend to be devoted to securing his/her position. Uneasiness will be disguised and energy will be devoted to thinking and feeling a way through his/her anxiety. The point at issue is whether the group members are going to be put off by a recognition of the anxieties of the leader, given that they might see the leadership as a source of strength. If it seems that they are not, then there is no reason beyond the fear of rejection why any groupworker may not make his/her apprehensions as much a point of discussion as the fears and expectations of everyone else, thus gaining credit for being human and adjusting the expectations of members to bring them much closer to the actual reality.

Such an action can be a mistake both in timing and in confidence if the leadership's assessment of the group situation is wrong. The group may actually be in a stage where they need to believe that they are led by experts. If so, then the disclosure of fallibility could be dangerous. But if it comes as part of the growing awareness between all members of the group, at a time when they are strong enough to realize that they are in fact working together, supporting each other and contributing to the group's life, it becomes an acceptable part of development.

Loss of control is a fear generated by an awareness on the part of a leader that s/he is at the beginning – that although s/he may have worked with many groups, the carry-over of skill and understanding is not precise; the process of growing into a group needs to be gone through afresh each time. The essential point of development is to recognize the symptoms and recollect the cause.

It should now be clear why this chapter is about responsibility. If you have conceptualized and created a group, then something which did not previously exist has come into being and you as convenor are responsible. If your aims are clear and you are going to direct what ensues from beginning to end, then there is no question that the overall responsibility stays with you. If, however, your aim is to enable your group members to take responsibility for their own behaviour and that of the group, then the responsibility issues become much less clear.

In so far as you are successful in generating responsibility in others, you then share responsibility with them while still maintaining any official responsibility as well as those of being an individual and a member of the group. While operating as guide, enabler, facilitator or whatever, you continue to exercise the responsibility consonant with that role. Thus until you withdraw entirely from the group, responsibility is part of the job. In fact, the responsibility entailed in the nurturing role is much more subtle and delicate than that seen in a directive role. Developing a sense of personal and group power in those who have ample reason to believe they had little requires leadership that is conscious of an enormous responsibility.

Most effective leaders adopt those areas of practice which are more compatible with their personality. In many cases this is a range rather than a precise point on the scale of the possible. Most also know that in any one group they may need to cover the whole width of the range at different times in the life of the group.

Stage-by-stage example

Stage 4: Intervention

As I have stated in general terms what kind of interventions were made in this group, I would now like to use illustrative material from the group to show different kinds of intervention.

Leader:	What did you do last week, B?
B:	I can't really remember very much. I know I asked how these group sessions were going to teach us more about groups than teach us about ourselves.
Leader:	What do you remember, J?
J:	Just that C talked a bit more and that S said that someone had got him down last term. I remember that.
	(Laughter)
Leader:	Do you know why you remembered that?
J:	Yes . . . No, I don't actually . . . Oh! probably because you asked me what S had said when he said it.
H:	I think we felt B would learn more about herself by our responses to what she was saying. That was the crux of the argument.
Leader:	Yes! What was your contribution then, H?
H:	Well . . . talking more about myself . . . perhaps more than I've done throughout the sessions we've had since the beginning of term.
Leader:	And you got a response?
H:	Yes.

I know that the recorded dialogue from a group is sometimes very hard to follow because all the behavioural factors which go to make it relevant are missing. But it is still quite easy to see that the leader in this recording is still the central figure through whom all interactions pass. This is typified by the question and answer nature of the dialogue. Nearly always, each person is drawn into the interchange by the leader. If this kind of intervention continued, then very little sense of being a part of the group would grow amongst the members, who would tend to feel that the power and domination rested with the leader alone. However, this came fom the early stages of the group when there was a great need, which the leader met, to get the group up and running and to make members used to the idea simply of being in the group and of contributing to it as they were able. The device of question and answer is one that they were all used to and it served to ease them gently into the group. Questions direct conversations, as they require answers. While they have the merit of keeping things going, they also have the disadvantage of ensuring that members do not contribute what is uppermost in their minds, but only what they deem might be an appropriate answer to the question.

In this next, very short extract from the group records it can be seen that the interaction is now between group members, and the leader's interventions are little different in kind from anyone else's because he is now much more going along with what is happening. The events in the group are going steadily towards the goal of learning about group processes and all he needs to do is interfere as little as possible, and only when the focus shifts for too long from the essential theme.

J:	Could you imagine me . . . if I was going it in the same situation and I couldn't do it either . . . just asking somebody. Is that clear? I suppose that's the obvious thing.
S:	Yes, but I wouldn't like . . .
J:	But I don't know why.
H:	Perhaps you were looking to P to put your ideas over a little more simply for the benefit of those who weren't understanding? So that you directed your comments to her for support, perhaps?
S:	No!
Leader:	That's three people I have heard to say that they are not getting much support from the rest of you in some way or other. I wonder why that is?
B:	I don't think I quite know why.
S:	I don't think I meant that.

119

WHERE RESPONSIBILITY LIES

Here the apparent coherence of the group has diminished, probably because they are thinking out the problem of mutual support for themselves. The leader's intervention is minimal and the question in his statement is open and not directive, more a kind of wondering than something requiring a direct answer as response.

Apart from anything else, this extract is a clear indication of the way in which people, when they become absorbed in some group issue, tend to pursue their own line of thinking in the presence of, but not necessarily with, others.

9

GOING ON, CHANGING DIRECTION OR ENDING

It must be apparent to all that some groups, having completed their tasks, actually come to an end. It must also be apparent that some groups come to an end before this point, for a whole variety of reasons. But what is less apparent but equally important is that some groups keep on going. Some continue in the same form as when they started. Others change quite dramatically, whether by an act of will of their members, by force of circumstances, or because they change what they are attempting to do.

Whichever of these positions a group holds, one of the essentials of good basic groupwork is that whenever members leave a group, what they have gained through membership should be as consolidated as is possible. The transfer of learning from a situation where it has taken place – and this is especially true of experiential learning, which is a major characteristic of group learning – to another, i.e. the ordinary circumstances of life, needs some essential back-up for its effects to be sustained when the support of the learning group is no longer available.

In one very important sense a group is designed to produce an end product, but in many cases that important and essential aim tends to get lost in the actual activity of creating and running the group. In this chapter I am going to try to make the case for considering the ongoing development of the group through to termination or transformation just as carefully as the group's conceptualization and setting up.

TERMINATION

Termination is, then, just as much a job which has to be organized as the more regarded one of setting up a group. In many ways it is actually the more difficult task because while there is the good feeling of having to create something from nothing in the initial stages of starting a group, there may well be some feeling of loss when the time for a group to end arrives. The feelings are, of course, largely controlled by whether the group is ending as a success in having achieved what it set out to do or whether it is a partial success or is ending dismally in some kind of failure.

121

One way of looking at this end stage of a group's life is to recognize that from the very moment of conception the group will actually have been working to this point. If a group has been set up to achieve a given goal or set of goals, then the point, distant in time, when it is achieved is also the point at which the group has no real reason for continuing its existence. However, there are many occasions in which a group in the process of attaining one goal discovers that there is some merit in creating others which can then be pursued. In other words, new contracts can be made as the group develops and begins to understand in a better or clearer way what it can achieve.

Of course, not every group which is established with a goal to achieve is able to achieve it successfully. Some goals are based on assessments made at the time of setting up which prove over time to be wrong. Such goals emerge as not within the capacity of the group, as constituted, to achieve. Many reasons may exist why a group cannot attain all of what it set out to do; examples include sickness, lack of resources, the existence of too many negative factors, etc. In that event it is the responsibility of the group leadership to make an assessment and to engage the group in a discussion of the group's continued viability. Ending a group has to be considered in various ways.

Open groups – that is, groups where the membership changes as members join and leave as they or the group consider they have gained what they can from attendance – never die. A club, for instance, stays in existence through many membership changes and finishes only when circumstances change so that no further members seem willing to join, or external factors operate to close it down. The issue of ending is therefore different and of a more personal nature in an open group than it is in a closed group, where ideally all members start and finish at the same time.

We will consider here various acts of termination, and the process of consolidation and the transfer of learning. In the next section we shall examine transformation as an alternative to termination. As always, we must consider the kind of assessment which is appropriate at this stage in the life of a group.

Assessment is fundamentally a matter of practical judgement. All leadership acts are based, or should be based, upon the judgement by the person making them that the act in question is a valid and probably necessary thing to do. This implies that judgements are the basis for all human actions, whether they are conscious judgements or not. Now this is far too wide a use of the word to be helpful in the present context, so that we must redefine assessment to mean a process by which a group member or leader becomes aware of taking stock of what is happening. This may start more from a feeling that there is a need to evaluate what is going on, or it may come from a fairly precise knowledge that some summing up of the group's progress is necessary to clarify for all where they have arrived.

The actual process of assessment may be done mentally and fed to the group in the form of 'this is what I see and think and feel is happening. What are your impressions of the situation?' This has the advantage that what any individual in the group thinks is occurring can be checked against how the situation appears to others. Even if this results in no overall consensus, it does at least make all members aware of the differences which exist in the group and realize the different impact which group events have had on members.

In effect, this kind of assessment should have been continuous throughout the group's life, as it forms the basis for all actions that members of the group and the leadership might take. It is also the basis of other forms of assessment in that the continuous stream of assessments eventually adds up to an evaluation of the total group judged against what it is trying to achieve. By recording the assessments which are made and comparing them with actual outcomes, the validity of any actions which have been taken can also be judged and the value of practice judgements checked.

To create a group takes a good deal of thought and preparation, and to end one takes much more of the same kind of consideration than is usually realized. Why? Well, in order for the gains which the group members have made to be retained, the period of termination has logically to include time to practise the transfer of knowledge, understanding and skill into the field of everyday life. Much of what has been gained in social treatment groups, for instance, can be lost if insufficient attention is given to consolidating gains before the members of the group are exposed to the pressures of life without the support of the group.

Thus the time of ending the group is concerned with assessing how valid such a procedure would be. Of course, if a contract has been in existence which stipulated a given time for ending the group, then any assessment must be one which has taken cognizance of this fact during the life of the group. Time, as we have seen, is one of the major constraints on a group, and assessment will naturally be largely concerned with establishing how much has been achieved in the allotted period and how best to ensure that those gains carry over when the group does actually finish.

Some groups do not achieve their objectives, as we have seen. Some might not succeed even if more time were devoted to them or a different approach tried, and thus the end of the group is brought about because assessment reveals these factors rather than any achievement. On the other hand, some groups achieve what they set out to do and then, having discovered what they can actually do and not being limited by time, set out upon another stage in their life. We will look at this later under the rubric of transformation.

A method which I frequently use in learning groups to bring about a constructive termination of the group is to set up a series of evaluation situations which culminate in the whole group pooling its information and sharing its learning. Such a group has a planned termination, and there will have been constant reference to the ending process during the group's life.

Example

A group which had been established to learn about the processes of groups and the ways that these could be used in helping situations had reached its final day. The group had been resident together for four days and had done some fairly intensive studying and working together. Now the leader asked the members to take time as individuals to make a detailed assessment of what they thought they had got out of the days they had spent together. These individual evaluations were then fed back to the members of the small work groups, and finally the shared material of these groups was fed back to the whole course. The similarities and differences were most rewarding, but above everything else was the sense that members had done everything in their power to integrate their learning before they left the group.

Clearly, assessment at this time is not just a matter of finding out what one has learned; it is much more concerned with sharing. But it is also concerned with a well-known but frequently ignored fact about learning, which is that often there is a difference between what one feels one knows and what one actually knows in hard, cold facts. In group learning this distinction is not quite so important, because one of the most fundamental aspects of the learning process in this case lies in the actual sense of having experienced being in a group and of watching things happen. Thus actual feelings are a very important part of the total learning that has taken place. Nevertheless, it helps very much to try to state what other kinds of learning have taken place, and it also helps others by emphasizing things they have learned and by reminding them of things they may have forgotten.

So much for a group which has a very definite time limit in which to achieve a given task and one which by definition would have to be a closed group. But what about a group which is going to go on for a long period of time and where the basic task is to exist for the benefit of the members? Such a group is by definition an open one, and termination applies to the membership of individuals rather than to the life of the group itself.

Example

The members of a psychiatric halfway hostel all formed part of a committee which administered the simple day-by-day routines of the hostel. This meant that each member was part of a very influential group which to a large extent controlled what could be done. Although each member also received attention from the psychiatrist and from social workers, discharge from the hostel and entry to it were matters for discussion amongst the total group. Jobs, which were allocated by the committee, sometimes meant that members ready for discharge would be asked to wait until a substitute could be found to do their task. The group as a whole were often faced with the task of coming to terms with the loss of old-established and very useful members of the community. Equally, they had to face the fact that new members would be arriving. A reception group was formed for this purpose.

In this situation the group was seen as an adaptation process for people who had been in-patients and who needed time and help to relocate and find accommodation and work, but did not need skilled nursing or medical care. As each person came into the group, which was relatively small, his/her needs as an individual were considered by the group. But the group's main concern was to initiate the new member into the life of the group. The hostel could function and provide a service only if it were to be a largely self-governing enterprise. Thus each new resident quickly came to recognize that his/her needs might be served only if the group were to be kept in existence by his/her efforts in combination with the efforts of others.

Termination in this kind of group meant that the period of adjustment to life outside an institution had been reasonably successful, that possibly work and some form of accommodation were available and that the support system of a self-help group had been substituted for the encapsulating care of a psychiatric unit.

Perhaps the most significant feature of all forms of termination in groups is that which is concerned with preparation. After all, when a person joins a group s/he has to go through the experience of being accepted, especially if that group is already well established, and of learning what the acceptable patterns of behaviour in the group are. Such a new entrant is concerned with whether s/he will be accepted by the group and also whether s/he wants to accept the group. Later that concern becomes less important and tends to be replaced by ones about the amount of influence the group can exert and about how much influence s/he wants and is able to wield in the group. Even later still, s/he may recognize that trust is an important part of group life, and the degree of liking s/he has for other members and they for him/her becomes important.

The whole of this process of working into and integrating with the group has to go into reverse when a member is leaving or when the group as a whole is closing down. The ties of liking need at least to be slackened and those with people outside the group re-established and/or strengthened. After all, these are going to be the relationships which will assume most importance in the future. Then the influence of the group has to be lessened also, but the learning which has taken place needs to have been as integrated as far as time and effort will allow so that it can be used without the support of the group. Finally, the actual presence of the member within the group will be terminated.

Group members carry with them the memory of their time in a group, especially if that time was either very good and helpful or very bad. When good, this acts as a reference group and serves as a storehouse of impressions and ideas, of feelings and of sources of behaviour. When bad, it tends to have the effect of making ex-members very wary of entering another group, however different.

It can be seen from this that I am advocating that as much care should be taken in ending a member's attachment to a group as was taken to establish it on arrival. Whatever the kind of group, if it had value for the member, then it is worth taking time and making an effort to ensure as far as possible that the value stays with the member after s/he has left. Too often, once the supportive ambience of the group has been given up and the care of the members and leadership left behind, the changes and the learning are seen not to have been well integrated into the personality and experience of the erstwhile group member, and the pressures of life can soon erode their effect.

Let us briefly recapitulate the main points of termination before looking at the idea of transformation.

Planned or unplanned termination

The ending of a group may be planned-in right from the group's inception; it is part of the original contract. If this is the case, then at various stages through the group's life progress towards termination should be assessed, and an essential part of the group's programme should be the working of all concerned to the point where the group ends.

Unplanned termination can come about through the fact that the group did not or could not include termination in its original planning because of uncertainty at the time. Unplanned endings also come about because the group cannot function effectively; because it cannot achieve what it set out to do; because members are being damaged in some way by the continuation of the group; or through such factors as loss of members or of leadership.

When an individual leaves the group

Individual members leaving from an open group generate a sense of loss in those remaining, and the whole process needs to be carefully worked through so that all understand the feelings which are generated. The consequences are different according to whether the decision by the group or the leadership that the member should go is intended to be for the benefit of the individual or for that of the group. In either case those consequences must be coped with. There is also the concomitant effect of the entrance of a new member. It must be remembered that the addition or loss of just one member can produce a much greater apparent disturbance in the relationships within the group than the mere numerical change would seem to indicate.

When the group as a whole ends

It is necessary that the preparation for the group's ending should be as effective as possible and links re-established with support elements outside the group.

The reactions of members

Even if a group has prepared well for its own ending there may be several members who are reluctant to go, especially if they feel that the group has proved very beneficial and supportive, and are somewhat worried about how they will cope without it. Alternatively, they may be pleased to go, having derived all they feel they can from the group, and be glad to reduce the commitment of time and energy which the group has demanded of them. In the former case members may attempt to delay proceedings by bringing up new ideas which they want considered and will present ideas for continuation, or, more usually, accepting that the group will actually end, producing the idea of reunions in the immediate future. Reactions may be quite diverse in that some members are more ready to go than others even though all are aware that the group has achieved most if not all of its objectives. There may also be some very strong feelings of loss if the group has been very cohesive and has become established in the members' minds as valuable.

The reactions of the leadership

Most of the reactions of the members may also be found in the leadership, for whom the group may have been a very rewarding experience.

The activities of the leadership in terminations

Of the numerous activities required of the leadership, the most important of all is the need for there to have been a constant assessment of the group's progress and that of the individual members. On this assessment can be based all the preparations for ending and the attempts to cope with the feelings which may be involved. These may range all the way from satisfaction with accomplishment to anger and reluctance. Regressive behaviour may set in, and delaying tactics on the part of those who are not entirely happy with the prospect of losing the support to which they have become accustomed over the life of the group. The group's achievements should be discussed, and how what has been gained can be projected into a future without the group. The process of cohesion which occurred at the beginning of the group should be reversed and the use of rituals like rites of passage employed or dramatizations of the process of change used. The leadership must also be aware that they too have to go through the same processes and feelings of loss or relief.

Consolidation of what has been gained should have an important place in leadership activities. This can be achieved by exercises with the group in assessing the facts of their progress and by clarifying from as many sources as possible what has been done. The whole purpose of the group may have been to bring about change, and if this aim has been achieved, then it is necessary to demonstrate and assert that it is so.

The transfer of learning is notoriously difficult because the support which made the learning possible in the first instance does not often exist when members leave the group and they are dependent upon their memories for most of the support they will need to sustain and integrate their newly acquired skills or knowledge. The methods of obtaining support from others and the use of recall should be discussed, with some illumination of the probable pitfalls and the signs that it is taking place.

Follow-up may be one way of helping the integration process, but the leadership have to be careful that this is not being used as a form of extension of the group's life.

TRANSFORMATION

Transformation has often been claimed as a new concept in the process of termination. But I am sure that many groups and workers have used some of the procedures which are listed under this rubric without actually being aware that they were doing anything different.

In essence, transformation occurs when a group decides that it does not want termination – that is, a complete ending of the group in its present form – but that it wishes to change either its form or its aims in some way, based on what it has learned in the process of developing. It is recommended that transformation should be considered as an option only if the group is already involved in the process of considering its own termination and provided that it has explored the process quite thoroughly. If at this point there is some consensus that termination is not attractive, then the exploration of alternatives can begin. This must not be a scheme to prolong the current existence. New group forms should be explored, the probability of resistance from some members and from leadership must be discussed, as too must the possibility that any new venture will split the group and cause resentment also.

There are several forms which a transformation can take. For instance, the group might continue in an attenuated form with meetings at more infrequent intervals, in essence becoming a form of follow-up. It can agree to be absorbed into a larger organization with similar aims; it can affiliate itself to other small groups working in the same area, as many issue groups have done, and eventually form a national organization of small cells; if it is a large group it can split into independent subgroups; it can set up its own follow-up operation or it can change its focus and continue with a different contract and different goals, which should be those which have emerged during the course of its life.

Whatever happens at the end of a group, it should be recognized that this is the point to which the group has been working ever since it was first formed, whether this was officially recorded or not. One of the main reasons why, although the effects of successful groups are frequently stable and enduring, they are not as stable as they might be is that while much attention is given to getting the group off the ground and in running it well, insufficient thought is given to the long-term effects. These are quite simply that where the group has achieved its purposes within the group structure and its lifetime, the most important element is that these effects should endure outside the group. It is to that end that more attention should be given to the process of termination.

Stage-by-stage example

Stage 5: Termination and assessment

The ending of this group of students had been fixed well in advance and coincided with the end of their academic course. So whether the group had achieved its task or not (or at least, whether it had achieved its task completely or only partially), it had to close down. Of course, this had some advantages and some disadvantages. When an end point is known so far in advance, it becomes part of the life of a group and defines the time available very precisely. This means that the pressure of time is always present and becomes a major part of the decision-making process, which might not have been so pressing had the group had unlimited time.

   The end of a group should see leadership acts becoming rather more prevalent than during the middle period as direction and support is given to the members towards being able to back away from the group and their involvement with it. This is the reverse of the starting moves, which were designed to bring the members closer together. In this student group the increase in the number of references to outside factors such as work situations was quite noticeable during the last sessions. There was also a great deal of effort put into discussing how they were going to use what they had learned about groups and about themselves. This involved trying on the role of leader of the group and attempting to produce given effects, e.g. controlling an animated discussion in a limited time span. Their efforts were later analysed by the whole group.

The main consideration, however, was what the job situations they were going back to would actually allow them to do. Although this is an eminently practical consideration and very logical, it also forms the basis of emotional withdrawal from the group in preparation for working outside it and without its help.

Alongside this consideration was another of almost equal importance, which was the attempt to assess exactly what each had got from the experience. This inevitably brought out some criticism of the leader, especially in those cases where members found that what they had got was not exactly what they had hoped to get, either in kind or in quality. I believe that whether such criticism is entirely justified or not, and it may well be that on most occasions it is, it forms part of the parting ceremony sparked off by some sense of loss, or probably of time not used to full advantage for any of several reasons. This becomes the time when the favourite phrase tends to be 'If only . . .', which seems to indicate a degree of regret for opportunities not taken.

It was interesting that during this period a fair amount of reference to the beginning of the group took place. For the first time, members felt that they could say clearly what they had felt about joining the group in the first instance and how anxious they had been. It emerged that most of them had been waiting for others to make the first move towards a better state of integration, a situation which often occurs and which can lead to stagnation and disappointment if it is not mitigated. The feeling that their behaviour had been superficial and cautious was put forward, and criticism of the leader for not recognizing their dilemma sooner and doing something about it was also advanced.

Because the group had spent some time working through the nature of its own ending, when the last group session occurred it ended in much the same way as all the others had done. Friendly goodbyes were said and some tentative arrangements made for future contact if and when it was needed after the course had finished. And then we all went our separate ways, feeling quite kindly disposed to each other, and it was all over.

Evaluating this group meant comparing it with dozens of others of a similar nature; taking into account what the members had said about it; and looking carefully at my records and at my own feelings. It had been a group which had been slow to develop trust, but this was not unusual. Several members had wanted to move at a much faster pace than others, again quite natural in such a group, but this is behaviour which tends to develop the braking power of the group rather than its accelerators. Finally, there was my own learning as leader and the mistakes I had made, which had been quite clearly outlined by the students in their comments, mainly to do with the assumptions I had made and with some lack of perception about some areas of this particular group.

At this point the cycle is complete.

10

THE DEVELOPMENT OF
KNOWLEDGE AND SKILL

If knowledge gets far ahead of being, it becomes theoretical
and abstract and inapplicable to life, or actually harmful,
because instead of serving life and helping people the better
to struggle with the difficulties they meet, it begins to
complicate man's life, brings new difficulties into it, new
troubles and calamities which were not there before.

P.D. Ouspensky, *In Search of the Miraculous*, 1950

There is no convincing evidence to show that teaching a pupil
about language does anything to improve his performance in
it. On the other hand, there is abundant evidence to show that
constant practice in talking and writing, especially where the
pupil's experience, interest and imagination are involved,
significantly improves performance.

R. Wilson in *The Criminal Survey*, vol. 5, 1971

By using these two quotations taken from very different sources I hope to
show that knowledge as a basis of practice has to be useful and adapted to
the needs of those who work with it. I also hope that the quoted remarks will
help to indicate that where a particular set of skills is required, then talking
about it is of little practical value in increasing the ability to perform.

If one substitutes 'learner' for 'pupil' in the Wilson quotation and 'groupwork' for 'language', the analogy is more or less complete. Both are practical
skills, both require creative practice. Groupwork may be considered to be a
more complex form of social behaviour than speaking a language, so there is
the danger that it will therefore be subjected to much more teaching *about*.

Groupworkers, like everyone else, need to learn their trade, and without
any doubt the best way of doing this is in a kind of apprenticeship situation.
No one ever truly learned how to operate in a group situation by reading a
book, no matter how good or how well written. Therefore all potential groupworkers have to face the situation that they will have to undergo some form

of supervised experience with an experienced groupworker who, if they are fortunate, will also be an experienced teacher.

The purpose of this chapter is to try to give some simple guidelines to the learning process, which otherwise can get very complicated, especially when it is realized that the main way of teaching people about groups revolves round their being able to analyse the dynamics of a group of which they are members. To put it another way, the learner has to be able to divide his/her thought processes, being able to be an active and participating member of a group and at the same time an impartial observer of the forces within the group which are affecting him/her and all the other members. It is not surprising that many people find this rather daunting, if not impossible. However, as the ability to function as a group member as well as be the observer is absolutely essential to being a good group leader, there is no other satisfactory way around this problem.

As we have seen, there are a great many different kinds of groups run by people with very different theoretical understandings of the human condition. But basically all groups have the same fundamental properties – that is, they all develop what we have called their 'processes'. The difference between groups lies in which of these processes the group's leadership and members choose to emphasize or diminish or ignore and which style of leadership is most compatible with the leadership's theoretical orientation.

Thus the first problem a beginner faces is whether to commit him/herself to one kind of groupwork approach or another. The choice of mentor will in fact mean that this choice has probably been made, for the style of the teacher/supervisor will most certainly have a lasting effect upon the student. This situation has other complications, not least the fact that apart from any theoretical orientation most practitioners have developed an individualistic style honed over the years to suit their personality and with which they have grown comfortable. Some, for instance, are only prepared to work with the individual in the group situation using the group as context.

However, before we start to look at what kind of group may be available for the learner to take on, it is necessary to make a passing reference to the problem of learning itself.

The first of these concerns an attitude which tends to prevail with regard to what might loosely be called 'social skills learning'. By this I mean all those areas of understanding of, and working with, people. It appears that many people believe that because they have achieved whatever age they have without major catastrophe, they are therefore 'by the light of nature' experts, or at least competent, in human relationships. This 'natural' approach to learning about human behaviour makes life for the teacher very complicated. Why? Well, for two principal reasons. If everyone actually learns all their coping skills in a 'natural' way, then any teaching about them tends to be regarded as artificial and 'unnatural', and hence is resisted. Second, what has been called intuitive psychology, which is another way of saying learning naturally, is often very prescient about some areas of human behaviour, if not in others.

But such social skills and learning acquired 'naturally' are at best what might be called 'parochial' – that is, that even when good they refer to, and are appropriate for, the limited and local situations in which they were acquired. This will be less the case if the individuals concerned have had wide experience of other ways of living and have had to adapt to a number of different social situations. The argument can be continued along the lines that if the natural processes of learning social skills are really as effective as some people seem to think, why have we got so many problems of relationships? The answer can only be found in the fact that so-called 'natural' learning in this area is adequate only for limited situations.

It is essential that this point be understood, because if it is not, what really requires a very serious study in order to be effective will receive only cursory attention. So we can say that learning about group behaviour and acquiring the skills of working with groups, or even of being a good group member, requires a great deal of hard work and a willingness to learn and to acquire skills. A great deal has been discovered about the way people behave, but hardly any of it seems to be consciously and widely applied to improve the lot of those who come into groupwork. What is required is encouragement to make an adjustment of beliefs to overcome the resistance to learning about human behaviour.

Effective groupwork is, above everything else, concerned with the ability to see what is going on in a group – in a word with observation. If a group leader is not able to see what is going on under his/her very nose, then there is no way s/he can be expected to do anything about it. It is always a pre-condition of action that, under normal circumstances, the person who makes it is aware that some kind of action is necessary. Such an individual may of course be wrong, but at least s/he has a perception of the situation which indicates the desirability of some form of action. Without this perception nothing will be done.

Western society does not approve of staring; it tends to embarrass people and is generally taken as being rude or offensive. But if we are to see what people are doing, then there is no substitute for staring, and staring hard. It is a truism of life that there is a great deal of difference between looking and seeing. For most of our daily lives we look at things, but we rarely see them, in the sense that if we are asked to describe them later we usually have only the vaguest knowledge of what was there. It is essentially a question of how much attention is paid to what is around us. The monitoring of what we pay attention to helps us to concentrate on those things which are of immediate importance and to screen out those myriads of impressions which would only confuse the issue and which are not seen as being either dangerous or relevant in some other way. If we were to pay equal attention to all the impressions which our senses offer us, we would, I think, soon become incapable of any form of existence.

So when we say that the first requisite of learning about groups is to watch what groups do, we are faced with the possible inhibition which society imposes on such activity. After all, group behaviour is not usually classed as a spectator sport. Any programme designed to help individuals become aware of group processes has therefore to build in some form of exercise which will free people from this embarrassment. It will have to give permission for individuals to stare.

The third learning difficulty is concerned with the fact that understanding of group processes is usually obtained by experiencing at first hand what those processes can do. In other words, one has to feel what they can do by being the object upon which the processes are working. Thus it is of little practical value to know that groups apply pressure to their members to conform, if one has not felt what such pressure is actually like.

Thus to recapitulate the three major learning problems:

1   There is resistance to the idea that social skills can be, or need to be, learned.
2   There is resistance to the idea that observation of others is an essential part of learning about behaviour, because of the in-built sense of embarrassment.
3   There is the need to recognize that experience of what the quality of group pressure is like has to be personal, so that some idea of its possible effects on others can be gained.

Of course, almost any group will do as a source of interaction which can be observed, but, as I hope to show, special exercises and involvement are necessary to be able to understand the other factors involved.

Given that the necessity of learning about human behaviour has been accepted, then the first point which has to be made is that of recognizing the way in which the group is effective in influencing the behaviour of its members. This can be done by a fairly careful analysis of any group of which one is a member, say a family or a friendship group, but it must be one in which the basic requirement for influence is fulfilled – that is, that we have a reasonably strong desire to be accepted as a member of the group. Remember, it is generally accepted that the greater the need an individual has of being accepted by any particular group, the greater the pressure that group can exert on that individual unless there are known and acceptable alternatives.

When one starts to look at the influence which groups have in this way, a strange new world can emerge. Actions which we would once have unhesitatingly accepted as deriving from personal initiative are now seen to be at least partly influenced by the effects we anticipate they will have on the group. The network of influence is seen to spread very wide indeed and to cover a great part of our lives. Let us just take one very illuminating example, the way decisions are made in a group.

Very often people can be heard to say that a group made some decision or other. Now I maintain that this is not correct. No group ever made a decision. What usually happens is that the group as a whole, or some major part of it, agrees to accept some point put forward by an individual. This implies that the group has ratified the proposal made by one of its members. Much has to be learned about the way in which decision-making procedures are affected by individuals, and also how they are arrived at, because lack of positive disagreement is usually taken as consent. This being so, one can say that any member of a group who disagrees with a group decision after it has been made has only him/herself to blame. Unless s/he was the subject of a deliberate campaign to exclude him/her, s/he should have realized that opposition to a proposal can be effective only if it is made plain that it exists. This applies equally to all other kinds of feelings that members may have and seems to be one of the hardest lessons that group members have to learn. It is no good assuming that other members in the group will recognize your feelings in some telepathic way; there is no neon sign which lights up with a message. What you feel, has to be made explicit so that other members are left in no doubt what you feel and are not then given to making assumptions or taking your feelings for granted. In this way the overall opinion of the group as a unit may be expected to be arrived at.

One very simple way in which the problems of decision-making in a group can be made clear to people learning about group behaviour is to set a group of learners a task which is (a) time-limited, and (b) requires the co-operation of all the members of the group to perform. If someone who is not a member of the group can be put in as a non-participating observer, so much the better. Because of the time factor, which puts pressure on the group to complete the task, many facets of group behaviour emerge: for instance, who will recognize the limitation under which the group has been placed, who offers suggestions, how roles are allocated and who assumes leadership and attempts to direct the group. When such a group is asked to report back on how they achieved or did not achieve their task, one fact becomes immediately obvious, and that is that because they were involved in doing something, they usually have only the vaguest notion of how what they did was achieved. This is where the observer comes in. This individual can feed back to the members of the group a fairly impartial account of what was seen, by virtue of the fact that s/he was not directly involved in the task the group was attempting to perform. When this impartial report is checked against what the members remember of their behaviour, some startling contrasts are likely to appear.

Certain members will most usually be seen to have taken control of the situation and have manipulated it to a given end, although this may not have been obvious at the time to those involved. Such individuals are people who from past experience and/or inclination have fulfilled the three necessary preconditions for making a leadership act:

1   They have recognized that something needed to be done.
2   They have felt that they possessed the resources and the desire to do it.
3   They have felt that it was worth the risk.

The task in such an exercise is often of marginal importance, but it does help if it can be something which the participants see as being either useful or amusing. I have frequently used the idea of the group casting themselves in a small drama about some well-defined theme or have asked them to prepare a brief requesting financial assistance for some project from an organization which requires the information immediately. Now, games these may be, but these exercises and others like them begin to develop skills which are essential to the use and understanding of group behaviour, and each participant experiences the learning they embody as a personal fact.

Take for example the act of decision-making, which we have just been looking at. It is essential than any group leadership should be able to recognize this process when it occurs; s/he should also be able to see which members are affecting the process and in what direction, with what intent and to what extent. Given that the leadership can do this, then the decision of whether to intervene in the process or not, at what level and with what intent, can be made.

Films of group actions and video tapes are very useful here because the action of the group can be played over and over again in order to show exactly what happened. Indeed, audio tapes can be used just as well wherever a one-way screen is available, and are another way of keeping a record of what is going on, though they have the defect of not being able to provide an action replay, merely the sound. There are some ethical objections to this process, particularly if the group being observed are unaware of the fact.

Video tape is widely used and is a very useful medium in the process of learning about group behaviour. But for me it has several drawbacks which reduce its practical value quite considerably. However well equipped the studio, there is no way that I have discovered which actually allows the recorder to cover the total interaction of the group without being so far away that the resulting film is almost useless for learning purposes. When groups sit or operate in a circle, which is a formation with considerable practical advantages, it is inevitable that some members will have their backs to the camera. If several cameras are used in an attempt to overcome this problem, the mixing of the shots from the various cameras becomes crucial and must flow with the action in the group.

Just take the fact that it is customary for individuals in a conversation to control the flow of who speaks with what emphasis by eye contact; the non-verbal clues which are set up by gestures all add to the richness of the communication. But in order to know what is going on in a group, a good group leader needs to know not just what the speaker of the moment is doing but how *all* the other members are receiving the messages being put out. It is

137

hardly possible to record all this wealth of detail on a tape, even with all the most up-to-date contrivances of split screens. It boils down to the fact that what ultimately appears on the tape is selective and edited, and with that we have to be content, even though we know that it does not represent by any means the full complexity of the interaction patterns which even a very simple group provides.

Such tapes are, however, of inestimable value in showing group learners more or less how they appear to others. There is a very short time immediately after the first experience of seeing oneself on tape for the individual to grasp the difference of expected appearance from what actually appears, before that window of opportunity is closed, as the mind seems to reassert the expected appearance very quickly. Many people these days have lost even that small learning opportunity through having become accustomed to seeing themselves on camcorder takes.

Audio recordings can be used to help group members analyse the group process in wide sweeps rather than in terms of individual contribution and immediate interaction. What the group as a whole is doing as opposed to what individual members are saying sometimes emerges very clearly from a sound recording. But all the non-verbal clues, apart from tone of voice, are missing, and the exercise is time-consuming in that each tape takes as long to listen to as it did to record in the first place. However, such tapes are very useful in showing the different styles of contribution to the group, especially in terms of timing and frequency and quality of intervention, etc.

Exercises in designing groups can be created from actual situations. For instance, a group problem can be set along the lines of 'This is the environment in which this group works; these are the known constraints; these are the known qualities of the group's members; the problems they face and the difficulties are roughly like this; these are the known resources and facilities available . . . now design a programme for this group which will best enable it to achieve what you think it is capable of achieving.' This is an academic exercise, but at least it encourages people to see the conceptualization stage of groupwork as of vital importance and tends to help individual learners avoid some of the commoner errors that occur in the setting up of groups.

Most of what we have looked at so far has been concerned with a group of learners in the kind of position where they can use their own group as a major instrument in the process of learning. But apart from being able to attend a groupwork course where this formation is a basic, most learners have to contend with learning a great deal in other sorts of situations. By far the best of these is a simple apprenticeship with an experienced group leader who is willing and able to instruct.

Such a situation can exist in a form of the co-leader situation which we discussed earlier. Here the learner has an accepted role in the group and is not seen as an intruder with an individual agenda which is not necessarily part of the group's programme. S/he can watch and participate, get feedback from the group on performance, and discuss with the experienced leader what was going on and what the effect of the use of certain strategies had been – in other words, be in a position to get first-hand experience both of being in a group and of being coached in the processes and techniques of leadership. Any discussion which follows working in the group is then based on recent experience and does not have the disadvantage of being somewhat removed from actuality, which is the bane of the more academic studies of leadership activities.

All potential leaders of groups should, if at all possible, have some experience of being a member of a group. If this can be as a member of a group where the essential purpose of the leadership is to instruct the group members in the working of the group, so much the better. As things happen in such a group, the leadership is going to make a point of asking, 'What do you see/feel is happening now?', constantly drawing members' attention to the prime purpose of the group when they are likely to have become involved in participation in its activities. This has some disadvantages, of course, for each time the leadership draws members' awareness to the processes of the group, there is the danger of disturbing the flow of those processes and of introducing a strong sense of artificiality into the proceedings. However, as the group proceeds and other members can take up the idea of examining what is going on, then the purpose of the group will tend to switch to the process of learning by self-examination and the sense of artificiality will begin to disappear. A whole series of enquiring and valuable leader and member habits will have started to become established in the members.

Perhaps the only real way in which one can realize what is happening in a group is to keep some form of diary. In too many instances groupworkers are prone to consider that an individual group session is the important factor in understanding groups. But this has been proven time and again to be not true. Groups exist in a time scale which can range from just one session to sessions lasting months, and even years in the case of treatment groups. The whole idea fostered by the idea of group development, however caused, is that any group session is influenced markedly by any sessions which precede it, and even to some lesser degree by those sessions which are due to follow. Given the fallibility of memory often pressed by events other than the group itself, what is recalled from one session to another is remarkably fragmentary, selective and nearly always out of sequence. Some form of recording is therefore essential if the large patterns which are synonymous with what we have called the group processes are to be seen emerging from the welter of individual session activities. Patterns of events will only be seen to emerge in their rightful context and with appropriate relationship to the group's progress if they are recorded with as much help as can be obtained from all sources involved as soon as possible after each session. The effectiveness of decisions taken and interventions made will then show up in ways that are not available close to the time when they occurred.

Of course, the way the group deals with its individual members and how they cope and change with the group is of paramount importance, but no one will ever see how those changes are being brought about if the larger patterns within the group are not revealed. Indeed, I have often heard groupworkers attribute individual change within their groups to what, after research, turned out to be almost wholly spurious reasons. If a group is being run with a co-leader, then one leader can assume some responsibility for recording while the other is concerned with the practical issues of leadership. If these roles are taken in turn, then valuable experience of being in the group and of watching for the large moves which are being made can be obtained. The great benefit for each comes when they share their experience at the end of the group while making the recording.

An essential source of understanding what is happening in a group is the feedback it is possible to get from the members. Sometimes this is done by questionnaire. But however it is done, it has two very distinct advantages: it indicates to the members that this is their group and their opinions about how it is working are of great value, and it also spreads the views to a wider ambit. For instance, when as an opening gambit in a session the members are asked to recall what happened in the last group, several interesting points emerge. What each individual remembers best is what more or less immediately concerned him/her at the time; taken altogether, a whole group recall constitutes a much fuller record of what actually happened. The weakest point of all recalls is the sequence in which group events actually occurred. This latter point is important. In pursuance of establishing the cause and effect sequence it is essential to get it right or the true reasons and patterns will be skewed.

A training programme designed to help people understand how groups operate is difficult to plan effectively. It has to start from what those involved already know or think they know about groups and also from what they have heard, thought and felt about any groups with which they may have been in contact. There has been so much written about certain kinds of groups that it would be very unusual indeed if some member of a collection of group-work students had not got some ideas about groups. These experiences and understandings will condition the approach an individual will make to any new group experience and will certainly influence both the quality of any learning and the preferences which will govern it. It is necessary to get across an understanding that learning to be a groupworker is not the same as, say, studying economics, because there is a direct involvement of the person both in the learning and in the execution of what is learned.

If at all possible, the feelings which individuals have about groups should be brought out into the open where they can be discussed and their influence on the ability of the learner to learn studied. In itself, clearing expectations and feelings like this can be a good example of how a group might operate to reveal individual agendas and is a process which is essential for some groups to function. Clearly, if the process is well done, then each member of the learning group will have not only a better chance to learn but also the sense that this was achieved in co-operation with the leadership and the other members of the group. The whole basis of group success – shared experience and resources – has already started to operate.

A most effective method of teaching in the group situation is by example – that is, offering a role model. If the leader is a good one, then because most inexperienced group members need some markers of what constitutes acceptable behaviour, they will tend to take their cues from the leader's behaviour. Thus a leader can consciously and deliberately influence the way members will go by displaying those behaviour patterns which s/he has reason to believe from past experience will be most beneficial. There is some considerable evidence to indicate that behaviour is seen, by those seeking reassurance as to how to act, as a more reliable guide than the spoken word. Whatever the leadership says should be done, if it is not seen to be being done, then not only is confusion introduced but the membership have every reason to believe that their leaders are being devious, and suspicion will develop because, particularly in the early stages of a group, members are almost always uncertain and self-security is important. If, for instance, a leader demonstrates that s/he cannot accept comment on his/her performance from members, then it is not very likely that the members will be prepared to accept any comments given to them about their performance by the leadership.

This is a very important part of the learning situation and one which many find very hard to accept. All that we know about non-verbal communication would tend to confirm that where anxiety and strangeness and maybe even resentment combine to make people feel that they are not as secure as they would like to be – that is, in a new learning situation where they are going to be exposed to new ideas and perhaps have their behaviour exposed to scrutiny – they become sensitive to the behaviour of others. In particular, they are sensitive to the behaviour of those whom they have reason to regard as possessing power and some experience – those who are seen as knowledgeable and able to influence the situation.

Anyone learning about groupwork needs to be able to practise what has been learned. There is a great need for learners to have the opportunity to take over existing groups and to try to exercise leadership; to try to guide groups; to try to adapt their behaviour to the perceived needs of the group and to obtain feedback from the group's members as to how they felt they were being 'handled'. It is essential that trainees should practise different styles of leadership no matter how much they feel that one particular style is suitable for their personality. It is not always possible or even desirable that a group leader should have just one approach; there should be some flexibility so as to be able to adapt in order to meet the group's needs at different times in different ways. All leaders should have the chance to be directive, for the beginnings of any group place great demands for security and assurance on any leader and it is well to be able to give it when it is required. Of course, some forms of group demand this kind of certainty in approach for the whole of their existence.

Role-play sessions and simulated situations can be an excellent way of providing a kind of trial run for those who want to feel what it is like to be in a leadership position before they actually have to play that role in a serious situation and have to become involved with others who may, for a time anyway, be very dependent upon their skill.

Books and other written material are the sources of ideas and approaches; of records of the ways in which others have tackled similar problems; and of the theoretical ideas which are available about groups and groupwork. The translation of ideas into practice, as we have seen earlier, requires different skills from those required to produce the ideas themselves, and not infrequently ideas have to be modified in practice to fit the situations in which it is intended they should be used. Much information is of a very general nature, more in the way of guidelines than of explicit rules of practice. Thus when in reply to my question to a groupworker, 'How are you going to cope with this?' s/he produces the answer, 'I don't know!', then the way is open to discuss what information is relevant. The difficulty has been exposed and the immediate value of appropriate information is recognized. Such information will most certainly become the property of the user, especially if it works well.

Learning about how groups operate is a special form of learning in that the groups which are formed to do the learning are encouraged to study their own behaviour in the knowledge that it represents the basics of what happens in all other groups except in the matter of selective emphasis. This latter fact can obscure what is going on for some people. I am thinking of those whose ideas of learning cannot so readily be adapted to this kind of approach because they seem to see that all groups are different and pursue different purposes in different ways, or because self-examination does not come easily to them. When the subject of one's field of study is people and their behaviour, then not only is one surrounded by one's subject matter but one is also part of it. There is no shortage of material; all that is needed is a little experienced guidance as to what is of prime importance to start with.

A final word. I have attempted to set down as clearly as possible and to enumerate the different ways in which the principal groupwork tasks may be undertaken. It has always seemed to me that this has been and still is one of the areas of greatest confusion for those interested in working with groups: the fact that there is little help in the literature in choosing between the various presentations and theories. The student is confronted with the need either to accept a particular approach backed by particular theories or to follow the precepts of a particular profession dealing with specific problems. This continues to lead to the inappropriate use of groups by a process of fitting the customers to a group form instead of the other way round.

Certainly approaches to groups have become more pragmatic since *Basic*

Groupwork was first written, and the degree of certainty with which one could write about things like the selection of group members has been diminished by experience and the realization that many groups contain members who have been selected by processes other than those a groupworker would normally use. This has had the effect that groupworkers have had to enhance their skills in working with groups which had a much greater pre-formed state than in earlier times, and to forgo many of the advantages which could accrue from selection.

I have tried to show that groupwork is an active and interventionist skill no matter how determined one may be to be otherwise. The very presence of a groupworker in any group has certain interventionist qualities. A newly created group is an entity which did not exist before someone set it up. It has to be guided in its progress by some form of direction, however discreetly and democratically, but guided it will be or it will disintegrate.

I suppose I must yet again stress that all groups of people behave in fundamentally the same ways. The major differences which appear in groups come from the different emphases of the belief systems and desires of their members and the objectives and theoretical assumptions of their leaders. This has a lot to do with the composition of the group and the varying strands of ideas and beliefs which are introduced into it from different sections of the community. But the assumption of the formation of processes in all groups makes it possible to learn about these basic elements and the uses to which they can be put without having to be anything other than a pragmatist.

The best way to learn about groups, as I have consistently averred, is to become an apprentice to some worker with considerable experience and, if possible, good teaching skills as well. Most of what is written in the groupwork literature takes on new and clearer meaning when it is read during and after experience within a group. There is no substitute for integrated and ordered experience, if only to learn the difference between the beneficial aspects of groups and their destructive ones. Knowledge itself is neutral; what matters is the use to which it is put.

FURTHER READING
AND REFERENCES

FURTHER READING

This list has been kept very short. Inclusion of a text is based upon the work being relevant, useful and easily available. Many references to other texts are to be found in the bibliographies of the books listed here, and also in the professional journals of social work, groupwork, psychology, sociology and education.

Brown, A. (1992) *Groupwork*, 3rd edition, Aldershot, UK: Ashgate.
Douglas, T. (1995) *Survival in Groups*, Buckingham, UK: Open University Press.
Douglas, T. (1995) *Scapegoats: Transferring Blame*, London: Routledge.
Mullender, A. and Ward, D. (1991) *Self-directed Groupwork*, London: Whiting & Birch.
Preston-Shoot, M. (1987) *Effective Groupwork*, London: Macmillan.

REFERENCES

Ahmad, B. (1990) *Black Perspectives in Social Work*, Venture Press.
Dawkins, R. (1989) *The Selfish Gene*, Oxford: Oxford University Press.
Douglas, T. (1983) *Groups: Understanding People Gathered Together*, London: Tavistock.
Douglas, T. (1995) *Scapegoats: Transferring Blame*, London: Routledge.
Goffman, E. (1971) *The Presentation of Self in Everyday Life*, Harmondsworth: Penguin.
Heap, K. (1968) 'The social groupworker as "Central Person"', *British Quarterly Journal of Social Work* 25(1): 20–29.
Lavoie, F., Borkman, T. and Gidron, B (eds) (1994) *Self-Help and Mutual Aid Groups: International and Multicultural Perspectives*, New York: Haworth Press.
Pinker, S. (1997) *How the Mind Works*, London: Penguin.

INDEX